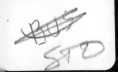

CHILDREN, PARENTS, LOLLIPOPS:
TALES OF PEDIATRICS

By

VLADIMIR TSESIS, M.D.

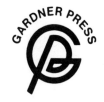

GARDNER PRESS, INC.
Lake Worth, Florida

Distributed exclusively by:
Paul & Company   Gardner Press, Inc.
P.O. Box 442   6801 Lake Worth Road, #104
Concord, MA 01742   Lake Worth, Florida 33467

Library of Congress Cataloging-in-Publication Data

Tsesis, Vladimir A.
    Children, parents, lollipops: Tales of pediatrics / by Vladimir A. Tsesis.
    p. cm.
    ISBN 0-89876-214-6
    1. Pediatrics—Popular works. 2. Pediatrics—Miscellanea.
I. Title.
RJ61.T87 1995   95-5801
618.2—dc20   CIP

Design & Typesetting by Artworx

9 8 7 6 5 4 3 2

TO MY WIFE, MARINA,
AND FOR SASHA

ACKNOWLEDGMENTS

FIRST I AM deeply grateful to my wonderful patients, their parents and families. They trusted and inspired me, they shared their hopes and doubts, their triumphs and failures with me. To them I owe an infinite debt.

Thanks to the wonderful staff with whom I was privileged to work: to receptionists Barbara Costo, Edith Ortiz, to medical assistants, former Russian physicians, Pavel Orlov, Polina Blyakhman, Irine Fedorova, and, especially, to my devoted partner, Doctor Meer Nisengolts. These people generously and faithfully helped me to carry out my professional duties towards patients.

Special thanks to my copyeditors Christina Sullivan and Betty Moore.

I am indebted to Gardner Spungin and Robert Paul for their friendship and encouragement.

I acknowledge my son Alexander ("Sasha") for his constant love and support. He read and critiqued various chapters of the book.

Finally, I would like to acknowledge the invaluable assistance of my best friend and partner in life, Marina. Without her extraordinary support and encouragement, this book could not have been completed.

Contents

CONTENTS

CONTENTS

CONTENTS

CONTENTS

Every man's life is a fairy-tale written by God's fingers.

—Hans Christian Andersen

INTRODUCTION

My decision to write this book was made after I attended an international seminar on medical ethics in San Francisco several years ago. During an intermission I spoke to Sara, a nice-looking young intern with freckled face, about her plans for the future.

"I would like to become a pediatrician," she told me, "but my father, an internist, tells me that along with the advantages of being a pediatrician come some serious disadvantages: long hours, night calls, and, especially, dealing with the parents of patients. Would you recommend that I become a pediatrician?" she asked me earnestly. "Of course, I would strongly recommend that you become a pediatrician. Just the fact that you are interested in medical ethics suggests that you are not just concerned with the monetary rewards of medicine or the technical side of medical practice, but that you are also interested in the art of medicine. There is no other branch of medicine that offers you more opportunity to enjoy observing the greatest mystery of life—the birth and development of human beings and their individual personalities.

"No other specialty in medicine allows you to receive such a moral satisfaction as pediatrics. In pediatrics you can give so much good to other people and feel good about your work and yourself.

"Working as a pediatrician allows you to be constantly in the invisible, powerful rays of life that emanate from children; you will not only work—you will be an active participant in the lives of many people as well. Therefore, whether in the office, at the hospital, or in your home your workday will not be filled with time-wasting, mundane, busywork; it will instead be filled with tasks that genuinely allow you to help other people, thereby giving you the chance to live a fuller and more meaningful life as well.

"To be a busy practicing pediatrician does not necessarily mean that you have to be a toiler in the field of health, but it means that you have a special lifestyle. This lifestyle might, during some periods, leave you exhausted, stressed out, and exasperated, but it also gives your life an additional quality. Your life is inevitably tremendously enriched by the experience of observing the lives and destinies of many people who, whether they know it or not and whether they want it or not, become a part of your extended and constantly increasing family. As a pediatrician, you are given the opportunity to actually perform good deeds, instead of just paying lip service to your desire and good intentions to help humanity."

"It sounds good," Sara answered, "but it's all just words, words, words. It would be easier for me to understand if you gave me specific examples from your practice that could illustrate your point."

"Examples!" I exclaimed so loudly that the people around turned to stare at me. "A thousand and one examples could confirm my words. In each day of my work as a pediatrician I observe and participate in situations that are more interesting than the most amazing stories you could read in any book. Let me think of which story I should tell first."

I wanted to start my first story, but the moment I wanted to tell it, another, more interesting and persuasive story would come to mind. Meanwhile, the light in the hall dimmed. It was time for the last session of the seminar to start.

"I'm sorry," I said, "we don't have time for me to tell my stories. Later, if you want, I can talk with you."

"What a pity; I'm leaving in two hours," Sara answered. "But I have an idea. Why don't you write one or two stories and send them to me. Here's my address."

I promised not to forget Sara's request, and once I returned home, I started to write my first story for her, then another one, and another until I realized that these stories should be compiled in a book.

This is not a book of advice and how-to. These topics have already been well covered by such authors as Drs. Benjamin Spock and Michael Rothenberg, T. Berry Brazelton, and Burton Schmitt. This book is about the life of a pediatrician and his patients, about their joy and pain, their ups and downs.

INTRODUCTION

One of the many benefits of being a pediatrician is having the opportunity to observe people as they really are in the "flesh and blood", not through the prism of the double-blind studies of medical research where the human soul is removed from the results during the process of the investigation, and the human being is reduced to columns of digits. Instead of this abstract generalization of a person, primary physicians see their patients in their wholeness.

The primary care physician, a pediatrician, who has contact with patients and their families for a substantial period of time has the chance to discover in each of these people the shining beauty of good decisions and kind actions of which every person is potentially capable.

Without this chance to see the best in human beings, it would be impossible for me or any other physician to stay optimistic and positive about life; sometimes you have to see the best if you are also going to have to see the worst in people. Without this optimism, how could anyone function after a patient becomes victim to one of the many heartbreaking tragedies of our fragile human existence? The testimonies of devotional love—indeed, the imitation of God—that the majority of parents demonstrate toward their children are this force that gives me the ability and the desire to continue my work after one of my innocent little patients becomes prey to death or an incurable disease.

Dealing with a child not only as a patient but also as a person helps a pediatrician become a part of the flowing river of life—life with its constant stories, the content and complexity of which are many times more fantastical and unreal than the most sophisticated science-fiction novel. The setting for these stories is the pediatric office, the hospital, and the doctor's home, and the actors are the doctor and the children and the adults who grant this doctor the privilege of practicing the best occupation existing to my knowledge—pediatric medicine.

1

THE JOY OF PEDIATRICS

I believe that individuals are predestined for certain life events. The way I became a pediatrician may have looked like a sheer accident—but this is another story—this accident, however, suited me like the design from above that I believe it was. On looking back over my long and still ongoing pediatric career that I began in 1964, I discover that I am happy to be a pediatrician. I consider this profession one of the most meaningful I could have entered. Not many professions offer such a wonderful opportunity to observe a human being who is growing, developing, and changing from visit to visit.

Though I know all of the drawbacks to my profession, they do not diminish my belief that the many years I have spent working as a pediatrician not only have been spent in the pursuit of a livelihood but have also allowed me to change things in this world for the better. It is one thing to theorize about helping people, especially children, and another to have an opportunity to really do it.

General pediatricians treat not a specific organ or a group of organs but the entire human being; the science and the art of medicine are harmoniously balanced. A pediatrician is a participant in the evolving development of human characters, lives, and destinies.

The work of pediatricians is frequently fraught with long hours, sleepless nights, and heavy responsibilities. Less frequently it involves unhappy, annoyed parents, managing the care of very sick children, and sometimes, sadly, the death of a child the pediatrician has known from the moment he uttered his first cry.

While physicians who specialize in internal medicine frequently treat conditions that are chronic and, on many occasions, caused or exacerbated by the patients' bad habits (e.g., alcohol and tobacco, overeating, a sedentary lifestyle), the pediatrician deals mostly with acute conditions that are treatable and preventable. Due to the acute nature of childhood diseases, one happy feature of pediatrics is seeing patients who were very sick become alert, active, and full of the joy of life—sometimes on the very next day after treatment—endowing all around them with their charming, angelic smile.

One of the worst aspects of being a physician is being an eyewitness and participant in the unending tragedy of human life—the suffering and death of patients. The pediatrician, however, has far less contact with this unhappy reality. Patients usually leave their pediatrician because they grow up or move away.

Pediatricians have the daily opportunity to witness the birth of intelligence in young children whose health, life, and destinies become entwined with their own. Pediatricians live in the midst of the great mystery of life, in a world of unending youth and development. Pediatrics is a constant reminder of the unconquerable dance of life.

Although I like children of all ages, most of the satisfaction I receive in my job comes from looking at children in their first two years of life, the years of divine innocence. No words can describe the delight of holding an infant, an entire human being who smiles a toothless grin at the doctor while the doctor makes sure that the patient is healthy and strong. All children are beautiful, but the age that intrigues me most is between eight and ten months. Observing children of that age, I sometimes have a religious feeling: it is not the sight of these wonderful children, that fascinates me, but almost a tangible sensation of a soul of a particular child that before my eyes has been transformed from an invisible, nonexistent state only several months ago—an instant of time—to the status of a real human personality, a unique individual entering in his or her innocence into a new, unknown world. I cannot think of many other professions in which one is surrounded every day by such beauty—an unfolding mystery of creation—and obtains so much aesthetic pleasure; amazingly, not only is all of this beauty of the emerging human personality free to the pediatrician, but parents pay the pediatrician for his services as well.

In this chapter I share some stories wherein my heroes—my patients—have given me some unforgettable memories. Other stories are about times when I felt I could make a difference by being there.

MY FRIEND LUELLA'S KOALA BEAR

ONE STORY that is very dear to my heart involves my seven-year-old patient Luella Calero. After I had treated Luella for a nonserious acute blood disorder her mother brought her to my office for a follow-up blood test. Luella hated fingersticks and did not disguise her resentment of them. Like many other children (and adults), she hated having any medical procedures performed and allowed me to do the necessary procedures only under protest. Though it appeared that Luella was sincerely trying to be cooperative, the moment the procedure began, she became resentful and unruly. She lay quietly on the examining table until a medical assistant tried to puncture her finger with a lancet, at which point she began yelling, crying, and struggling in order to avoid the procedure. It took two medical assistants and me, using all forms of persuasion—as well as physical restraint—to prevent Luella from jumping off the examining table.

When the procedure was over, I offered Luella a lollipop; she took it without even looking at me and only after some moments of hesitation. She obviously had serious doubts about the sincerity of my intentions. As she hesitantly reached out for the lollipop, I noticed a little clip-on koala bear toy clamped on a pocket of her T-shirt. The koala was very cute, and I asked Mrs. Calero where she had gotten it. I was not sure Luella was in any mood to talk with me. She told me that Luella herself had brought the clip-on toy home. Having no choice, I directed my question to Luella. Showing no emotion, she told me that she had traded her Barbie doll for the toy. I complimented her on her fine clip-on toy again, and we parted.

I had known Luella since soon after her birth at Bergler Memorial Hospital. I met Luella's father that day in the hospital, but he disappeared from the family not long afterward. Mary Calero had not handled her husband's departure very well. She had a horrible time dealing with the reality of becoming a single mother and felt lost without the support of her spouse.

Mary lost at least fifty pounds, becoming very thin. An anxious expression became a constant feature on her face. Six months after her husband left, she was hospitalized for treatment of severe depression. I was told all of this by Mary's parents, who brought Luella in for her medical exams during this period. Fortunately, the treatment of Mary's depression was successful. After six months she was released from the hospital and has been fine ever since. Now, seven years later, she held a steady, white-collar job. Her face was still young and attractive, and only traces of that anxious expression remained, unnoticeable to those who had not known her during the most unhappy period of her life.

Two weeks later Mary brought Luella in again for her regular complete blood count test. Surprisingly, Luella, who was still wearing her koala bear clip-on toy clamped to her T-shirt pocket, took the impending procedure with less resentment than in the first visit. Perhaps by now she realized that the procedure was good for her and was, at any rate, unavoidable. Even the procedure itself took only a moment because Luella was much more cooperative, though the expression on her face was far from contented.

At the end of a visit, I usually ask the people who have accompanied the young patient if they have any more questions. When I asked this question of Mary, she answered that she was worried that Luella might have streptococcal tonsillitis. She was running a mild fever and had complained of sore throat early in the morning. Looking attentively at Luella's throat, I could not see any change in the appearance of her tonsillitis but, despite my reassurance, Mary remained unconvinced. "Then," I told Mary, realizing how negatively Luella might react to such a recommendation, "we will have to check her throat culture to make sure she does not have streptococcal tonsillitis. The results will be available right away."

I left the room and went to see another patient, but in a few minutes I heard loud noises. A battle was going on between Luella and the medical assistants, who, with her mother, were trying to talk her into allowing a swab to be taken from her throat. I went back into Luella's examining room and found her in the middle of a fight. As she had during the blood tests, she again responded reasonably to our explanations, but when it was time to take the throat culture, she once again began to resist, crying and screaming, "No tests, no tests!" Her slim body writhed like a snake, and she used her fingernails as a defensive weapon against the medical assistants as they tried to restrain her.

At last, after several minutes of suggestion and a slight amount of physical effort the assistants succeeded in taking the throat culture. Though the objective had been achieved, I felt disappointed and regretted that we had not found a more peaceful way to deal with Luella.

In a couple of minutes, I returned to the Caleros with the good news: the throat culture results were negative, as expected. Mary was happy to hear that her daughter was not suffering from streptococcal infection. I started to write a note in Luella's chart. A minute passed before I realized that someone was standing next to me; I raised my eyes and saw Luella. She was looking at me, holding something tightly in her right hand. Before I could ask her what she wanted, she extended her arm toward me and opened her hand. In it I saw the wonderful koala bear clip-on toy, that I had admired.

"Here, Doctor Tsesis, I want you to keep it," she said in carefully articulated speech. She put the toy on the desk in front of me and, without another word, went back to her chair.

It was very hard for me to believe that this girl who, minutes before, had been so unruly, immature, violent, and uncooperative was now giving me a present of respect and understanding, a present more precious to me than all the gold in the world. Instead of holding a grudge against me—the person who, for reasons that might not be quite clear to her, had put her through these procedures, Luella had found enough maturity in her young heart not only for forgiveness but even for kindness and generosity.

I suddenly felt overwhelmed by my feelings. Here in my office I had witnessed the nobility of a human being, the kindness and capacity for forgiveness that were possible even in a young child. I realized that Luella's inappropriate response to the procedures was generated only by her uncontrollable fear, a response that she would eventually outgrow, as have many other children I have seen who had similar reactions.

I then gave Luella my present: an inexpensive electronic watch, which she accepted with dignity and gratitude.

Mary told me she was not surprised that Luella had behaved in this generous fashion and added with a happy smile, much like the one I had seen on her face the first time we met nine years ago, that Luella "is always like that."

"She gave it to you," she told me with pride, "so that the other children who do not have such a koala bear toy might see it."

I fulfilled Luella's wish by regularly wearing the dazzling koala bear toy on my stethoscope. When I am asked where I got such a clip-on toy, I respond, "I got it from a child who was very kind and generous."

TARANTELLA

Everything passes and vanishes;
Everything leaves its trace;
—William Allingham, *Blackberries.*

PASQUALE GRIPPO was an eleven-year-old child who was developmentally disabled. He was brought to my office by his parents, who had come from Cleveland, Ohio, for a month-long visit with relatives who lived in a Chicago suburb.

Pasquale had developed an ear infection, and this made him more disorganized than usual. As I began the exam, he was unruly and uncooperative, constantly moving, waving his arms and legs, and ignoring all his parents, admonishments for good behavior. He refused to sit up. His attempts to flop backward and lie down on the examining table were prevented by his father, who caught him each time he flung himself back.

Of the many ways to relax a child and make the medical environment less intimidating, one of the oldest and most effective is music. To entertain Pasquale and to see his reaction, I started to sing the uplifting melody of "Tarantella" to him. To enhance the melody of "Tarantella," I began snapping my fingers as an accompaniment to its fluctuating rhythm. Alas, my patient did not react positively to my performance—there was no happy expression on his face. He did, at least, stop falling into his father's hands and began producing some poorly articulated sounds, periodically looking at me with some degree of interest. I did not give up; I finished the "Tarantella" refrain and shook hands with my still poorly cooperating patient.

The next time I saw Pasquale was two weeks later for a follow-up visit. He looked quite different from the way he had looked the first time I saw him. He was studying a book that his mother was holding for him; there was an expression of great concentration on his face. On seeing me, Pasquale broke into a wide smile. The gloomy and uncooperative Pasquale that I had known from the previous visit now became animated, laughing so much that I had to ask him to contain his ebullience for the time being so that I could complete my exam.

Sensing my pleasure in observing his improved health since the previous visit, Pasquale became even more inspired. "Doc, Doc," he said to me, and then suddenly I heard him humming the melody of "Tarantella." The next thing I knew he was snapping his long fingers to the rhythm of the melody as an Eastern European would. I was not surprised to hear the melody from Pasquale, as he could have learned this melody from his Italian family, but this finger-snapping he must have learned from me.

EVERYTHING LEAVES ITS TRACE

PEDIATRICIANS ARE, by definition, "Baby Doctors," but actually, babies make up only half of their business. The other half is the care providers: parents, grandparents, aunts, uncles, and so on, and this group frequently presents the major challenge. Pediatricians might choose to spend their career complaining that their patients' caregivers were abusing them or could, instead, try to gain wisdom from these challenging encounters, thus accumulating a lifetime of experience that only medical practice, not theory, could provide. This experience not only can be applied not only to a successful career but also gives one interesting insights into human nature.

I cannot help but be amazed at the scope of human characters, the difference in the temperaments and attitudes of people belonging not only to the same community but often to the same family.

It took me many years to understand that when someone speaks to me in a rude manner, it might be only a mask for that person's insecurity. In addition, some people, although they are by nature nice people, may sound rude and lack manners because of their poor education. This does not on any account mean that I advocate rudeness and a lack of civility. It only means that not all aggressive reactions are really meant to be aggressive and that before I react with resentment, I usually try to give the other party the benefit of the doubt.

It was difficult to do this when Thelma Hardy brought her three-years-old daughter Agatha, who had been a patient of mine since her birth, for a mild infection, at the base of the nail on her left thumb. To make sure there was no hidden underlying infection, I carefully inspected the area of inflammation but could not see an abscess forming or any other signs of an active infection. To be on the safe side, I prescribed antibiotics and warm soaks for Agatha's hand.

One morning, a week after I received a call from Ms. Hardy at the office. Without introduction and in a loud, impolite manner she told me that her daughter's condition had worsened after some initial improvement. When I asked her why she hadn't brought Agatha in for her follow-up visit, she replied to me that, being on public aid, she could not always afford the cost of transportation to my office. On this day, however, she would be able to get a ride as her boyfriend was not working and could drive her.

I did not want to tell Ms. Hardy that she had been impolite; there was a more important issue to solve—I was worried about Agatha's thumb. First things first.

An hour later Ms. Hardy was in the office with her daughter. On examination I noticed that the small area of inflammation had become larger. An abscess was now forming on Agatha's thumb.

After minor surgery—incision and drainage—that I performed in the office, the pus from the abscess was removed, and I then put a dressing on the wound and wrote a prescription for an oral antibiotic. I asked Ms. Hardy to take Agatha to a nearby hospital's laboratory for a complete blood count to see how her system was reacting to the infection.

Although I had written a note on the laboratory request form that I was to be called as soon as the results were available, many hours passed, and I had still not heard from the lab. At four o'clock I was nearly ready to leave the office, and I called the lab to get Agatha's results. I was surprised to hear from their receptionist that Agatha had not yet come to the lab for her tests. Concerned that something could have happened to the family, I called Ms. Hardy's home to make sure that everything was all right.

I decided at this point that if Thelma was at home and continued to be impolite and coarse with me I would advise her to look for another pediatrician. But where had she disappeared to? The phone rang for more than two minutes; I was ready to hang up when someone answered. It was not Thelma but her mother, who also lived in the house with Thelma, Agatha, and Thelma's boyfriend.

On hearing my concern for her granddaughter's whereabouts, the grandmother, in an unexpectedly friendly manner, told me that I shouldn't worry. Her daughter had not gone to the laboratory earlier because she had decided to do some work around the house first. Fifteen minutes before my call Thelma and Agatha had gone to the laboratory.

Satisfied that at least the lost was found but unhappy that my request to have the tests performed as soon as possible had not been taken seriously, I thanked the grandmother and was ready to hang up when I heard a laugh on the other end of the line.

The office was closing so I had time enough to ask the grandmother the reason for this unexpected reaction.

"You probably do not remember me, Doctor, but I remember you well. My name is Carol. I took Todd, my other grandson, into your office for an exam two years ago, and thanks to what you said to me then, I stopped smoking."

Intrigued, I asked her to remind me what exactly I had said two years ago to produce such a powerful effect so that the next time I would know the magic formula.

"No problem," answered Carol, who now spoke to me like a long-time friend. "Though I am not as young as I used to be, I still remember things pretty well. You told me, 'Carol, you are such a wonderful woman. Please, for my sake, stop smoking to save your precious health and live to be 100 years old.'"

"Is that all I told you?"

"That's all. Nothing else. For sure."

"Then, I made a mistake. I should have told you to live not to 100, but 120 years, Grandma Carol."

Carol had a good sense of humor and answered my joke with a burst of youthful laughter.

A COMPLIMENT

PHARMACEUTICAL COMPANIES in the United States, in their struggle to gain new markets, are generous about distributing their new and old products to doctors' offices. Sometimes the amounts in the samples are more than generous. Not wanting to be used by big business, I put their generosity to a good purpose: for those patients who have limited means, the sample medications I am able to provide help them save a little on health care.

Mrs. Sofie Zenfield, the mother of four children, was very grateful to me when I gave her free medicine for the treatment of her daughter's ear infection. She left the examining room holding onto her daughter with one hand, her other hand filled with boxes of medicine.

When I came out to the waiting room to call the next patient, I observed that Mrs. Zenfield was speaking with the parent of a long-established patient, Mrs. White, whom she knew as a neighbor.

"You see," she said with satisfaction, "Doctor Tsesis gave me all this medicine. He saved me so much money!"

Mrs. White was definitely in a good mood on this day. "Oh, he is so sweet!" she responded with enthusiasm, turning her face toward me and giving me a big smile.

At this moment I wished it were always so easy to garner a compliment.

BRAVE FOREVER

ONE REQUISITE for being a pediatrician is the ability to cope with crying children. The most frequent reason children cry during an exam is, of course, the injections that are "generously" given in a pediatric office.

To prevent an unpleasant outburst on the part of my four-year-old patient Jay Chandler, I asked him, half in jest, whether he was big and old enough to no longer be afraid of shots. If he had answered in the negative I had some techniques to persuade him not to be afraid. To my surprise, however, Jay not only responded with a forceful "Yes" but was energetically nodding his head as well.

My surprise at such a strong reaction was noted by his mother, Dorothy. "How could you forget that!" she said to me. "Remember, two years ago when he got his vaccinations you were so impressed with his courage that at the end of the visit you gave him a card—a note that you wrote with a fine gold marker. It read, 'I do not cry when I get shots.' Since then he is never afraid to get his shots."

ENLIGHTENMENT

Mrs. Grace Phillips, a librarian, had been coming with her children to my office for the last ten years. Nowadays with divorce being so common, I had not even realized that she had been divorced from her first husband, had happily remarried, and now had a healthy four-year-old daughter, Yvette, from the second union.

Her children from the first marriage, Lesa and Joy, had grown up and rarely came to the office. I hardly recognized Grace's eighteen-year-old daughter, Lesa—a nice, good-looking teenager—when she came into the office with her mother for a potentially serious problem. Lesa had "lost her pep for life," which could be a sign of depression, and when I looked at her, I saw that she was telling the truth.

After an interview with Lesa and her mother, I came to the conclusion that the reasons for her problem were most likely of an emotional nature. From what I could see, the main cause was, that Grace thought of her as an adult and therefore spent very little time with her. Lesa continued to live at home, and her basic needs of food, clothing, and shelter were being provided, but emotionally she was on her own. Another contributing problem was Lesa's recent unresolved conflict with her now ex-boyfriend.

I was encouraged, however, that my patient was sincerely trying to find ways out of her predicament. We had a long conference and discussed some possible solutions to Lesa's depression. It appeared that Lesa was quite receptive to my suggestions; however, because of the potential danger of her state of mind, I told Mrs. Phillips that it might be helpful for Lesa to consult a psychiatrist or a psychologist.

A week later I received a letter from a psychiatrist, Dr. Gordon, in which he confirmed my impression of Lesa's condition. Dr. Gordon also wrote that Lesa had chosen not to proceed with psychiatric treatment, believing that she could solve her problems by herself.

I did not see Lesa in my office since that visit, but her mother came once in a while with Yvette. When I asked about Lesa, Grace, a sincere and open woman, would simply tell me that she was doing well after the first and only conference with me. I did not want to press her for more details, thinking that she would talk about her older daughter if she needed to.

A year passed after I had my long talk with Lesa; as usual it was Yvette who came to me for a visit with her mother. The day was not busy, for once I did not feel tired, and Grace was in good spirits; again I asked about Lesa, and again Grace told me that she was doing well.

"Come on, Grace," I said, only for the sake of Lesa, in the hope that she really had been able by herself to manage the depression that I had observed in the initial stages a year earlier, "you have told me she is doing well for a long time, but I want to hear more from you."

"What can I tell you? She and I are spending more time together—time that I set aside especially for her. She is doing really well—she made up with her boyfriend, and she is doing well at school and at work. She is really grateful to you."

I strongly doubted that my only talk with her older daughter could be so important as to effect this kind of improvement. "Why to me, Grace? In all honesty I should tell you that I did nothing special."

Though a pleasant smile remained on Grace's lips, her eyes took on a thoughtful expression.

"How can you say this! What you said then was more than important for us to hear," she said, not hiding in her voice her reproach for my skepticism.

I did not know how to answer her and was embarrassed by my own insensitivity. Seeing my embarrassment, Grace added, with a smile that people usually reserve for their most intimate friends, "Of course you did something special. How could you even doubt it! The reason this has upset me is that all this time I thought you knew how important what you said was for Lesa. What you said might be trivial and superficial for you, but for us it was a turning point."

TO THE WORLD OF SOUNDS

THOUGH MY partner, Meer Nisengolts, and I both emigrated from the former USSR—indeed, our accents betray our Russian backgrounds—we were unable to build a significant Russian clientele in our practice because of the location of our office. Most of the Russians who relocated in the Chicago area settled on the far north side, while our office is located on the west side. Thus, Russian-speaking patients who have reached our office are usually there for complicated problems that require good communication between doctor and patient, which is, of course, much easier when both parties speak the same language. I was, therefore, somewhat surprised to see on the chart of my new eight-year-old Russian patient, Yuri Friedman, a sticker written by a medical assistant that stated that this patient had come in for a simple checkup.

I entered the office and introduced myself both to the patient and to his mother. From the information in the patient's file I learned that Yuri's mother, Valentina Friedman, was a single mother. She had come to the United States about a year ago from Tashkent, the capital of Uzbekistan.

As soon as I began asking Valentina about Yuri's health history I saw that my new patient was not an exception to the complicated-cases rule. Indeed, a special condition had forced Valentina to bring Yuri on the long trip to our office. This condition was, without a doubt, Yuri's behavior. Something was definitely wrong with the way he conducted himself. Though he was dressed nicely, and his face was pleasant, with big, almond-shaped, coal-black eyes, he looked strange, as if he were not living in a tangible reality, but in another dimension of time and space. The assistant may have been right in writing that Yuri had come only for a checkup, but Yuri definitely had some medical condition that made him look as if he was off in the clouds.

Valentina, a woman in her late twenties, was big in all three dimensions, but her size did not interfere with the natural agility typical of people her age. She, her father, and her son shared a two-bedroom apartment in West Rogers Park, an area of Chicago where the majority of Russian immigrants settle when they first arrive in the United States. Though Ms. Friedman was working at her first job in this country, doing minimum-wage work, she was still far from fluent in English, and our conversation was only in Russian.

"Ms. Friedman, I know that you brought Yuri for a school physical, but I cannot help but notice his behavior. Why does he behave so unusually?" I inquired.

Valentina turned her face toward me. "My son behaves in the manner that is usual for him," she announced, giving me a brief look and then resuming her melancholic look at her son.

"Maybe so," I remarked, "but I have the impression that your son does not hear well."

"I know. My son is deaf and mute. I thought I had mentioned it to your medical assistant. He was born like that," stated Valentina, and she resumed looking at her son, who seemed to be running in all directions at the same time.

The more I observed Yuri, the more I realized that, deprived of appropriate stimulation from the outside world because of his deafness, he was trying to actively compensate for this void. Refusing to give up, he was filling the silent world around him with external stimuli of his own making. Paradoxically, though to the outside observer his activity might look chaotic, Yuri, flying like a butterfly from one object to another in the room, was consistently keeping his mother in his field of vision as if he were inviting her to participate in the hustle and bustle. Thus, Yuri was taking the initiative and was trying to engage Valentina in some form of communication that his mother did not know how to maintain.

Though the reality that Yuri created might appear to be artificial and distorted to those who were not living in his world of silence, he was trying to open a window to the world of sounds that surrounded him, rather than living in the world of deafening silence that was isolating him from other human beings.

Yuri's natural intelligence was propelling him, out of loneliness, to seek the warmth of human companionship, to seek partners in his exploration of the outside world. He was not only entertaining himself, but also trying to entertain his mother. Though Yuri's plea to his mother for nonverbal conversation was very obvious, it appeared that Valentina did not realize what her son's attempts were all about. I was amazed not only by Valentina's lack of reaction to her son's constructive efforts but also by the incredible energy that Yuri was expending out of his internal need to establish a bridge to the outside world. Despite Valentina's lack of awareness, there was no doubt in my mind that she loved her son—Yuri looked well cared for and was dressed in clothing that looked far more expensive than this family's budget would allow for.

Yuri was running here and there, all over the examining room, putting things together, only to scatter them a minute later as his fancy struck him. The more I watched Yuri, the more I felt that my notion that Valentina did not have a clear idea of how to handle her son was correct. Valentina's melancholy might easily be explained by her inability to interact constructively with her son despite Yuri's continual invitation for a nonverbal dialogue.

Trying to be as tactful as possible, I shared my observation with Valentina, who listened politely but showed no genuine interest. Her seeming indifference lasted until I asked her why she did not use sign language to communicate with her son. "I am too busy with my English classes to study sign language, but my son is learning it at school," she answered defensively, doing a poor job of hiding her feelings of guilt. Though she might have a good excuse for not learning sign language in her new country, the only possible excuse Valentina had for not learning it during the first seven years of her son's life in Tashkent—when there would have been ample opportunity to study sign language—was the irrational expectation of a miracle. I found out that, ignoring the medical prognosis that had no doubt been given by Yuri's doctors, Valentina had chosen to believe holistic healers and quacks who promised that eventually Yuri would hear. This advice had thereby absolved Valentina of the necessity of dealing with the problem.

Yuri was now in a really difficult predicament: in his own family the spoken language was Russian, and neither his mother nor his grandfather knew any sign language, while at his school, where he was beginning to learn sign language, the spoken language was English.

Though Yuri was silent, it was clear that his mind was filled with a noisy confusion of ideas. This was counterbalanced, however, by his inner need to find his way into the world of other people. He needed help.

I had no idea how to organize some practical help for my deaf and mute patient. Valentina told me that Yuri had just started a new school, and, thus, she did not know any of the teachers there. Generally speaking, Valentina's attitude to her son's possibilities in this new school might be as fatalistic—che sarà, sarà. She preferred not to speak too much about it and was not very receptive to my different suggestions. Though Ms. Friedman was trying to suggest to me that all she wanted was to get her school form and get the exams over with, I felt that on the subconscious level at least, she needed and wanted to know more about her son—otherwise why go to the trouble of traveling such a distance to my office? Some hope was there; I felt sure of it.

Though she listened to me with a detached expression on her face that bordered on rejection, I followed my own strategy and continued my discussion; I felt it was my obligation as a physician and as a human being to impart my ideas to this deaf child's mother of the possible techniques she could use to help her son merge with the real world—the world of sounds.

I asked Valentina whether she was aware of the laws in the United States that mandate that Yuri had the right to be educated like any other child, able-bodied or disabled—laws that must be followed by the school system. Valentina looked at me without expressing positive or negative emotions; she presented a picture of towering indifference. As a former immigrant, I understood her perfectly. In her look I could easily discern the skepticism of a person who once lived under the Soviet socialist system. Under this system the best laws and the best constitution existed on paper, but every Soviet citizen knew these to be only for show, only for the benefit of outsiders. Valentina assumed that here in the United States, the laws that were supposed to help her son were surely nothing more than a smoke screen for gullible, unsophisticated people. In Tashkent, where she had lived and worked as a poorly paid technician, she heard a lot of unfulfilled promises, which taught her to take life without forming any unrealistic expectations. Valentina's low expectations produced the apathy and lack of hope that were so eloquently written on her face.

Ignoring Valentina's impenetrable appearance, I continued to ask her questions about Yuri's old and new school, especially about the teachers at the new school.

"I don't know too much about Yuri's teachers, but there is a nurse at the school," Valentina said in a voice without inflection, as if she were simply yielding to my pressure. "Like you, she was asking me a lot of questions about my son. I can ask her to give you a call. Would you mind?"

I answered that I would be happy to talk with the nurse but even more with Valentina herself. At this moment, however, I felt that Valentina had lost interest in our conversation. Frustrated at my inability to help Yuri, I signed the school form and said good-bye to my unusual visitors.

Three days passed. I was told that I had a phone call from a woman named Pat Perelmuter. I tried but was unable to place her. When she come on the line, she explained that she was the nurse at Yuri's school, the one whom Valentina had mentioned during her visit to my office. Her voice seemed to belong to a woman of fifty years or older. Within the first minutes of our conversation I felt that Pat was sincerely interested in helping Yuri Friedman. She had called to ask my impressions of Yuri. She listened to my opinion with lively interest, interrupting me with many questions. It gave me much satisfaction to know that someone from a school system with a sophisticated crew of special education teachers, mental health workers, psychologists, and psychiatrists might still value the opinions and advice of a general pediatrician. I did not miss the opportunity to explain to Pat the psychological impact of being an immigrant.

I began to receive telephone calls from Pat on a regular basis. Soon I could easily discern her caring, gentle voice. During our telephone conferences I learned that Yuri was making progress in his struggle to "break the sound barrier." It is unfortunate that to this day I have never had the chance to meet Pat, but I am happy just to live in the same city where someone like Pat lives.

Valentina, Yuri, and Yuri's grandfather came to my office six months later. What I saw far exceeded any hopeful expectations I may have had when I first met Yuri and his mother. Valentina was like a woman who had been awakened after many years of being under a magic spell. She was vivacious, her eyes were full of life, she had lost at least thirty pounds, and on her face—oh, miracle—there was a sweet, gentle smile. I could barely recognize in this happy, energetic woman the dispassionate automaton I had met just six months earlier.

As if this were not enough, both Valentina and her father—a man in his sixties who looked like all good parents of the world—were able to maintain a conversation with Yuri in sign language!

Yuri had grown at least an inch, and, although he was filled with energy as on the first visit, it was no longer the chaotic energy of a flooding stream of water but was instead an energy that had been channeled and directed to purposeful, creative processes. His intellect had found an open window to the outside world, and he was taking real satisfaction in being a part of the events in it.

Astonished, I was unable to say a word, while Valentina beamed at me with a proud, maternal smile. She was right to be proud of the transformation that had taken place in her family.

"You see, Doctor Tsesis," Valentina told me in Russian, "it was hard for me to hear from you that for many years I was not doing all that was necessary for my son. Later I understood that you were doing it with the best intentions. You woke me up from my slumber. But, the main person who helped Yuri to achieve what you see now was, of course, Pat.

"Right, Yuri?" she asked her son, first aloud, and then, with an apologetic smile, she addressed her son in slow, but obviously precise, sign language, while Yuri attentively stared at her with his keenly penetrating and searching coal-black eyes.

He replied to Valentina in sign language, saying something that made Valentina smile.

"What did he say?" I asked.

"He said that Pat is his angel."

"He is right," I said. "Pat is a real angel for all she has done for your son."

"Well," said Valentina, and then paused. Not being a sophisticated woman who could easily express her feelings, she needed time to find the appropriate words. Her face blushed. Instead of the robotlike creature I had met a half a year earlier, before me stood an inspired and passionate woman. Though she was visibly embarrassed, she was committed to finishing what she wanted to say.

"But I also have *my* angel," she blurted out finally, and, looking straight into my eyes, she conveyed more than a thousand words could say. Indeed, silence is sometimes more eloquent than a million words.

At this moment I wished Helen Keller were alive to share with us the overwhelming feeling of being a part of the human race that, ultimately, speaks the same language and shares the same feelings.

A CHOO-CHOO TRAIN

ONE OF the qualities that distinguish a pediatric office from other medical offices is the noise level. It wouldn't surprise me if, during extraordinarily noisy moments, an outside observer got the impression that he or she was not in a doctor's office but in a slaughterhouse. Though over the years I have gotten used to children crying, I definitely prefer them to be happy and smiling. Ten years ago I began to transform my office from a dry, unfriendly place where children were brought against their will by their parents, to an environment where they felt themselves to be in their own "habitat." As an independent practitioner I was not constrained by needing the permission of all kinds of bosses, the approval of committees, or resolutions made by special panels; my only partner agreed with my inclination to make the office more fun. I went to many different stores, spent many long hours, and within five years my dream had come true: my office had become a "pediatric wonderland." Children and adults who visit the office now see the embodiment of my dream in the numerous toys and contraptions, that are placed unobtrusively all around. These toys can be turned on, lighted, and brought to life one by one, or all together, with the push of a button. On these moments I see, to my satisfaction, the same picture: surprised and excited little patients, wide-eyed and open-mouthed, observing one of the "thousand-and-one toys," installed in the office. Frequently the parents of the children display an even more spontaneous reaction of amazement; like their children, they do not expect that the toys and contraptions that were hardly visible before being turned on will come to life and begin jumping, running, spinning, and producing funny noises in such a prosaic place as a pediatric office.

Without a doubt the examining room most popular with the children is room number two, which features a choo-choo train running around the walls with an accompaniment of other toy trains, planes, battery-operated and remote-control toys, and colored lights. Many stories from this room of fun could be told; one of the most memorable and precious to me involved a young patient who was visiting his grandparents in Chicago when he became ill.

Gerald Roldan was nineteen months old; he was from Jacksonville, Florida, and was brought to my office by his maternal grandmother, Annette Kline. He came to my office for a condition that children his age frequently get: he had a viral infection of the upper respiratory tract that was complicated by a serious bilateral middle-ear infection. Mrs. Kline, a short, nicely dressed woman in her early sixties, was very helpful in providing me with a good history on my patient. She was taking care of her grandson while his parents were in Norway for the funeral of Gerald's paternal grandfather

Gerald's nose was very runny, his eyes were red and glassy, and his fever was 101°F. He was crying, irritable, and calling for his mother, as would the majority of children in his place. His grandmother was doing her best in trying to comfort him in his distress.

One of the critical moments of a pediatric visit is the ear examination. Frequently during this procedure a child needs to be restrained, especially if the child's ear canal is occluded by earwax. Though I perform this unpleasant procedure many times a day, as I examined Gerald I felt really sorry for him—only two days ago he was in his own sweet home with his parents and toys, and now, though under the faithful care of his grandmother, he was in another city and was sick, irritable, and tired.

To make his ear examination less traumatic, I decided to entertain him.

"Gerald, did you ever see a choo-choo train?" I asked him. Without waiting for his answer, I continued, "I am going to show you one."

"Choo-choo train," echoed Gerald unexpectedly.

"His father's hobby is miniature trains and Gerald has one of his own," his grandmother, Annette, explained to me.

"Where is choo-choo?" demanded Gerald of his grandmother.

At this point I turned off the lights in the room, and the shining fluorescent stars became visible on the ceiling; then I turned on a multicolored light projector that shone onto a revolving mirror ball. At the push of another button the many different toys came to life: a yellow pecking chicken, a monkey, a plane, a helicopter, and a rainbow-producing contraption. Another press of a button, and Arlo Guthrie's "The City of New Orleans," one of my favorite songs, started to play.

Finally, I turned on the transformer, and the train began to circle the room atop its continuous acrylic shelf. As Gerald looked at the toys, he forgot for the moment about his runny nose, painful ears, and illness. I saw that in the darkness of the room he was straining to catch a sight of the choo-choo train merrily running along the office walls. He stood up on the examining table and, pointing his tiny finger at the running train, smiled and repeated again and again, "Choo-choo train, choo-choo train."

Annette thanked me for entertaining Gerry when she left the office, and I soon forgot about the visit.

A month later I was somewhat perplexed when I received a small package from Florida, but the identity of the mysterious sender was easily resolved when I opened it. Enclosed was a picture of my now-healthy visitor, Gerald Roldan, playing with his own toy train, and a card from Gerald's parents thanking me for my special attention to their son. They asked me to accept their modest presents. Actually, these presents were not modest but were very precious to me. I still have them: a large ceramic cup with a train depicted on it and a T-shirt that has "Choo-Choo Train" printed on the front along with a splendid image of a toy train busily running forward toward a bright, yellow-red sunrise.

HOW TO GET A GOOD DISCOUNT FROM A CAR SALESMAN

THOUGH THE everyday practice of pediatrics might sometimes be burdensome and difficult, any pediatrician who has been in practice for a substantial amount of time would, on summing up his or her career, remember an extraordinary moment that overshadowed the drawbacks of the occupation and gave a satisfying notion of real achievement.

Things were routine one day when a nurse from Bergler Memorial Hospital called my office early in the evening to notify me of the birth of a female infant for whom I had been assigned to provide neonatology services. Though in instances where the newborn appears healthy, the accepted policy requires the physician who cares for a newborn child to perform the physical exam within the first twenty four hours of life, I prefer, when it is possible, to do such an exam as soon as I can. It seems to me that the parents who have waited patiently for the last forty weeks for their child are justifiably eager to be reassured that their child is healthy and strong once it has finally arrived.

As was usual for the autumn season, the office was quite busy, so I was unable to arrive at the newborn nursery until seven o'clock that evening.

My healthy patient, baby girl Grossman, was as handsome and lovely as any human newborn can be. The examination of the baby proceeded without a hitch; the baby was in good health.

I had decided to leave the examination of the baby's eyes until last since my attempts to do it at the beginning of the exam had been unsuccessful, because the baby wouldn't open her eyes. To examine a baby's eyes, the doctor shines light from a special instrument, an ophthalmoscope, into the newborn's eye; when looking through the ophthalmoscope, the doctor should see a red-light reflex from the retina. (This same red-light reflex that causes an infant's eyes to glow red in a photo, as many amateur photographers find to their dismay when they are taking pictures with an unsophisticated camera where the camera lens is located next to the camera's flash). The examination of a newborn's eyes can be a very quick procedure if the baby keeps the eyes open, but when the baby resists the procedure, and when his or her eyelids are puffy and swollen, and a sticky, slippery antibiotic ointment has been put into the eyes to prevent infections (and all of these problems are true of newborns), then this procedure can be more time-consuming, even when a nurse is doing her best to help "unlock" the baby's eyes. Unfortunately, baby girl Grossman presented all of these problems, and the exam had not been a piece of cake. Additionally, the nurse was busy with other pressing responsibilities and was not available to literally give me a hand with the examination. Holding the ophthalmoscope first in the left hand, then in the right hand while, at the same time trying with the other hand to open the slippery, puffy eyelids (and instead turning them inside out), I spent a substantial amount of time bustling around the crib where the baby lay until, at last, I was able to manage to see the pupil of the baby's left eye. As I expected, the red-light reflex reassured me that the eye was healthy and intact.

Then it was the right eye's turn. The light went through the pupil, but what followed was an unpleasant surprise. I checked my finding again and again, but instead of the red-eye reflex, the right eye of baby girl Grossman had only a thin, silverlike, bright shaft of light. It took me a long time and much rechecking, but I finally came to the conclusion that my finding was correct.

After I made a note on the baby's chart, it came time for the more difficult part of my visit; time to break the bad news to the parents of baby girl Grossman. Someone has to be the messenger of bad news. I entered the room with, as on many similar occasions previously, an unpleasant feeling. The Grossmans, who were alarmed by the long examination of their daughter, were impatiently waiting for me.

I felt very bad as I told the parents as delicately as possible of my findings, doing my best to reassure them that due to the early diagnosis and, therefore, the possibility of timely intervention, the prognosis for the baby's vision might be quite good.

Unfortunately, the Grossmans belonged to a sizable category of parents who, in order to accept an unpleasant fact, need to hear the same information repeated many times. Only at nine o'clock that evening, after having answered the last questions of the anxious parents, was I able to leave the hospital.

On the next day an ophthalmologist, Dr. Filtzer, called my office and confirmed that, indeed, there was a congenital cataract in baby Grossman's right eye. Though I was complimented by him for making an early diagnosis of the condition, which is usually diagnosed at a later time, I felt sorry for the baby, as the congenital cataract might permanently decrease the vision in her right eye. Congenital cataracts create a barrier to light that prevents the occipital area of the brain from receiving visual information, eventually leading to an irreversible dysfunction in the brain. Even if the infant's retina is intact when the cataract is later removed, the brain, which has been deprived of optical stimuli, is sometimes unable to recognize objects and, thus, is no longer able to process visual information. I hoped that eye surgery, which was already scheduled at Children's Memorial Hospital, would be successful.

I later learned that the Grossmans had named their daughter Abby. Abby never came to my office after she was discharged from the newborn nursery, as the Grossmans lived quite far from my office. My only source of information about Abby's condition was the letters from eye specialists that I received, initially on a regular basis and then less and less frequently. According to the letters, Abby was making steady progress. In a year my name was dropped from the mailing list, the letters stopped coming, and I heard no more about my patient.

I would never have been reminded of Abby Grossman if my wife, Marina, and I had not been shopping for a car some three years later.

After looking at some cars, we were sitting with a salesman in a poorly lighted corner of the store, discussing the advantages of different types of cars and unable to come to a decision.

At this moment the door that led to the business office opened, and a big, balding man in his early thirties came out holding a heavy briefcase in his hand. He almost passed us by, when, on seeing me, he stopped and began staring intently. His gaze was piercing, and he scrutinized me carefully. I waited patiently for an explanation, not having any idea why he was so interested in me. Marina and the salesman looked at both of us with curiosity.

"Are you Dr. Tsesis?" he finally asked me, and when I nodded in the affirmative suddenly a wide smile appeared on his face. He looked at our salesman and in a loud voice exclaimed, "Sam, do you remember I told you about the doctor who saved my younger daughter Abby's vision? That's him, Dr. Tsesis! Do me a big favor, Sam, give this guy a really good discount!"

SHARING LIFE'S BEST MOMENTS

AUDREY PORTOPILO was married to a local well-known businessman. She was a petit, pretty woman in her late thirties. Nowadays her natural beauty needed to be enhanced a bit by cosmetic means, which she used a bit more generously than might be expected, but I remember a time when, without any makeup she looked like a real queen. Audrey had long, naturally blond hair, and she liked to use bright red lipstick. She was a good mother, and for years she had come to my office on a regular basis with her three children.

Though Audrey appeared to be a happy person, she did not belong to the category of people who like to display their passions. The only two things she did with a real passion that I was aware of were child rearing and gum chewing.

Though her children were outstandingly well behaved, I never observed Audrey disciplining them; she was a mother who had a fine, natural sense of being both a parent and a friend to her children. Interestingly, as a rule, she was entertained by her well-behaved children, and not the other way around, as is usually the case during doctor visits.

Audrey never tried to impress our office personnel with her husband's position. While we were discussing issues related to her health insurance, I inadvertently found out that he was an important cog in the Republican machine.

On this day Audrey came to the office because her two-year-old son, Patrick, was complaining of an earache and sore throat. His case was very typical, and as I examined Patrick, I engaged in light conversation with his mother. Though Audrey was actively participating in the conversation, her appearance was different from the usual. She seemed to be concentrating on her own thoughts and distracted during our chat. In addition, her face, which usually wore the expression of a practical woman, instead radiated inspiration and quiet happiness.

After finishing Patrick's examination, I went to my desk to make a note in his chart and to write a prescription for him. My professional relationship with Audrey prevented me from asking her the reason for her sunshinelike appearance.

Patrick was my first patient on this not very busy morning, so I was in no hurry, and Audrey and I continued our conversation. We talked about children, education, health issues, and politics. For some reason Audrey was less and less interested in our dialogue—until finally, instead of looking in my direction, she began to stare at the wall across from her.

I blamed myself for my habit of sometimes being too informal with patients' parents and proceeded with the medical part of the visit, trying to stay away from any subjects unrelated to that.

The prescription had been written, and I was ready to hand it to Audrey when I noticed that her cheeks, which had been rosy from make-up before, now blushed a natural crimson.

As she took the prescription and during my explanation of how to give the medicine to Patrick she was still looking at the wall above my head.

I tried in vain to recall our short conversation, searching for a possible blunder on my part, when I noticed Audrey had turned her eyes to me as if she had come to some decision. Patrick was busily playing with a toy he had brought when Audrey asked me whether I had a minute for a private conversation. I was glad to be given a chance to discover the reason for her distracted mood and hoped that I had not said something inappropriate.

Mrs. Portopilo's beautiful dark brown eyes looked intently at me; I could see no enmity in them.

"Dr. Tsesis," she said, "I haven't told anyone about this yet."

What is this? I thought to myself. Am I in some soap opera?

"I haven't even told my husband yet," continued Audrey. At that moment I witnessed the most dramatic gesture I could have imagined from Mrs. Portopilo: she reached with her right hand into her mouth—carefully, so as not to smear her lipstick—removed her chewing gum, wrapped it in a tissue, and threw it into a wastebasket. My eyes were wide open. I was ready for a major surprise, and what I heard exceeded my wildest expectations.

"I wanted to tell you that I am pregnant. I just found out about it this morning, using one of those over-the-counter kits, which have always been accurate for me in the past. I can't wait to see my husband and tell him this news, but I had to share it right away, and I decided to share it with you!"

Before I had thought about it, we were embracing each other with a feeling of awe for the precious gift to mankind—the opportunity to have sons and daughters who can make the lives of their parents happy and meaningful.

The youngest child of the Portopilo family was born uneventfully in due time. He is a happy, plump baby with cheeks like two ripe peaches. Audrey brings him into the office for regular checkups. For me he is a precious reminder of what a privilege it is to work in a specialty where people share and entrust me with the most intimate secrets of the family, of which the most wonderful is the mystery of life.

2

SWEET EXPERIENCES

After I joined an existing pediatric practice and became a senior partner, I tried to eliminate two types of giveaways— little presents for our patients—that had become an established routine for the office. I was able to rid the office of bubble gum, but the popular demand for candy was so strong and pressing that we were forced to immediately resume supplying our patients with it, though we were well aware of the unacceptability of this sugary promoter of tooth decay in a pediatric office. My only consolation was that this candy giveaway ritual was practiced widely by many health professionals who deal with children.

From almost any child from two to sixteen (and older), a request for candy can be expected, and the most popular color of candy is red. Lollipops are also called "suckers" by my patients, who are unfamiliar with this word's other, well-known meaning. I never make jokes with this double entendre; my visitors, however, unhampered by my sense of professional restraint, do so from time to time. Recently, a young mother gave a lollipop to her impatient two-year-old daughter and said to her with a smile, "Here, have it—a sucker for a sucker."

A well-known theatrical critic once said that if there is a rifle hanging somewhere on a stage, it ought to be fired sometimes, meaning that every object around us should serve some purpose. Through the years sweets have unexpectedly come to serve me in my work as a pediatrician as more than just a small treat to give a child.

To anticipate my patients' requests, I sometimes ask a child whether he or she wants a piece of candy; as a rule I hear "Yes," pronounced in a thousand undescribable variations. After one memorable episode, however, I began preceding this question with a question to the parents on whether they mind if I offer candy to their child.

Mrs. Modena, whose husband I had never met, was a well-to-do mother. She had a pleasant face and a well-proportioned body. She was always very neatly and carefully dressed. I had seen Matthew professionally on a regular basis since his birth and can attest that Mrs. Modena took excellent care of her son. She breast-fed him for his first ten months and was very concerned about his well-being.

The most remarkable of Mrs. Modena's traits was her ability to look at me with a hypnotic, intent, and unblinking stare. I pride myself on my own ability to hypnotize people, but she easily beat me in my attempts to imitate her fixed, concentrated gaze. I always blinked first, though I must admit I never used all my talents in this ritual, not wanting to be discourteous to Mrs. Modena.

To solve this problem, I developed the habit of looking alternately into her unblinking eyes and then at her handsome child. Our conversations were always of a medical nature, never about personal matters, but it seemed to me that she liked me well enough as her son's pediatrician. I saw her child frequently, and she always seemed satisfied at the end of these visits.

Two and one-half years after I began treating Mrs. Modena's son, she became unhappy and openly irritated with me during a regular office visit. On this fateful day I, not realizing what I was doing, automatically opened a drawer and offered Matthew a piece of candy, forgetting that on one occasion Mrs. Modena had asked me in an emphatic tone not to give her son this treat. I realized my error when I heard the firm and unyielding tone of Mrs. Modena's voice, which was usually remarkably soft: "Please, do not give my child candy. I asked you once, didn't I?" I did not want to lose her son as a patient after three years of established relations and apologized as profusely as I could for not honoring her request. But looking into her fixed gaze, I saw no forgiveness; instead, I saw that the sentence was against me. Indeed, before a week passed, I received her request that I transfer her child's records to another pediatric office. As a result of this incident, we switched to sugarless candy, though on a special request, we can still produce politically incorrect lollipops.

This case was not at all typical; the overwhelming majority of parents overlook the undesirable effects of candy because of its one wonderful quality—giving their children a moment of pure happiness and satisfaction.

My professional resentment about this popular item changed to a feeling of tolerance after I discovered that a piece of candy sometimes helped me to look deeper into a child's personality.

For instance, when dealing with "difficult" children I have observed on many occasions that when they are made unhappy by shots or other medical procedures, they prefer to protect their infantile desire for omnipotence, and, thus, they refuse to take the sucker that is offered to them as a token of compensation for their good behavior. As a result the more energetically the lollipop is offered to these children, the more forceful is their rejection.

Brian Raffallo, a twenty-two-month-old prodigy, was brought in by his parents for a behavioral problem. The parents were worried that Brian had become too aggressive; he was hitting other children and even his mother and was experiencing visible pleasure from his "excesses." In the process of our hour-long conference, I observed that Brian easily and willingly accepted the piece of candy that I offered to him after some pretty intense psychological intervention, which included challenges to his feeling of omnipotence. Brian's desire to accept the little treat was one reason I predicted a quick and successful outcome to his problem; this prediction did come true.

As far as "normal" children are concerned, the "conscientious objection" to accepting sweet treats starts sometime around the age of six. Prior to that age a piece of candy can be used as the universal "bribe" for the young child.

There are exceptions. Martin Ferguson, a three-year-old marvel, on being asked, "Do you want some candy?" answered with a determined and forceful, "No." Seeing that I had an unusual "customer," I offered him stickers and other "valuable" goodies, only to hear the same resounding, "No!" After exhausting all the "prizes" I could think of to satisfy my picky patient, I inquired of him what he *would* like to receive.

"Give me the pink medicine!" Martin exclaimed, while his mother, who, on the way to my office, had been prepared for this energetic request, smiled broadly. "Pink medicine" is the common—though not yet accepted in the dictionary of children's slang—name for

Amoxicillin. This most commonly prescribed antibiotic in pediatric practice deserves its fame among our young clientele due to its appearance and pleasant taste.

I then asked Mrs. Ferguson to share a funny story of the day about her little genius. "Well, at three o'clock in the morning I was trying to give him some Tylenol for his fever when he taught me to be more precise about your instructions," she related to me. "When he saw me giving him his medicine from a tablespoon, he clenched my hand and lectured me, 'How come you are using a soup spoon? Didn't the doctor tell you to give me my medicine with a teaspoon!'"

In order to establish their autonomy, children learn how to manipulate their environment. Their pediatrician is included in this environment. Leroy Siem, a thirty-month-old youngster who expected generous compensation for his good behavior, addressed his mother in a voice loud enough for me to hear, "Does he know that I love the orange suckers best?"

Fedele Verni, a five-year-old tyke with black curly hair, coal black eyes, and a very healthy appearance, reminded me twice of my responsibility as a good citizen to be fair in distributing the "common goods." His mother was working, so he was brought to the office by his grandmother. Letting his grandmother know that he wanted to go home now and would like to complete the agenda of the visit, he pulled her arm and whispered loudly, demonstrating emphatically his impatience, "He always gives me a sucker!"

A month later he came in again, and the story was repeated. As his grandmother and I were finishing our conversation, Fedele openly criticized the insensitivity of his doctor, saying in a loud, passionate voice, "Where is the sucker!"

Lollipops have even helped me to discern abstract thinking development at an age when I did not suspect such thinking was possible. Clarence Kelly, a thirty-month-old, was brought by his parents for a well-baby visit, during which his immunizations needed to be updated. Near the end of the visit he received a piece of candy "for good behavior," which he took enthusiastically. At that moment a medical assistant came into the exam room, hiding in her pocket a syringe that contained a vaccine. When he saw the syringe come out, Clarence started to cry at the highest possible pitch and decibel level and threw the candy with all of his might at the desk where I was sitting.

His mother was laughing and trying to calm him at the same time. She turned to me and explained his reaction, "I told him, 'Clarence, for taking your shots you will get candy.' Now, with this behavior he is saying, 'Don't give me the shots. I'm not interested in your candy!'"

My experience with lollipops has also helped me to learn that children are incapable of the artful deception at which some adults are so adept. Of course, children are not saints—they do deceive, but they do it as charming amateurs.

I must confess that there was a time in my life when I began to feel that I was either a popular prophet or a rising political star. This usually happened at the end of an office visit when suddenly my desk would be surrounded by children who were devouring me with devoted, admiring eyes. Pleased by such an outpouring of feeling, I would stroke their hair and smile at them patronizingly and fix my tie—until a two-year-old boy peeped to me, "Sucker!" Alas, he let me know that I was respected not for my looks and personal qualities but for the sweets I could provide.

Two-year-old Richard Clements cried bitterly while looking at me, asking "Candy?" and then turning to his mother, pleading "Home?"

Three-year-old Dennis Hodges looked at me with reverence and deep respect, but I wanted him to speak and express his real wish. He, however, remained silent. "Do you want something, Dennis?" I inquired after accepting for some time his unblinking, flatteringly faithful stare at me. After a short pause, Dennis eventually betrayed himself, hissing energetically to me, "S-S-S-Sucker!"

Blanka Morales, three years old, did not give up her cherished silence as easily as Dennis. After I asked her whether she wanted something, she was silent but continued to look at me with deep concentration. Eventually I gave her an opportunity to save her honor by asking her, "Do you want a sucker?" With innate dignity she replied, "Yes, I'll take one."

Five-year-old Carl Brewer was not as proud. To his mother, who was asking her last questions at the end of a visit, he exclaimed reproachfully, "Hurry up, I want to have a lollipop!"

I conclude this tale of "sweet experiences" with the phrase that came from five-year-old Janel Young. When I handed him a big piece of candy, he looked at his mother and father with sparkling eyes and shouted victoriously, "That's what I came for. Candy!"

3

SPEAKING WITH PARENTS

I sometimes feel as if I have practiced pediatrics on two different planets. For the first ten years of my pediatric career I was in practice in the Soviet Union. My family and I emigrated to the United States in 1974, and by 1978 I had finished my pediatric residency in the United States and passed my examinations, after which I resumed my career in children's health care.

I had a difficult time finding work in a private practice after my residency in the United States, as most pediatricians in established practices prefer partners who have done their schooling in this country. Thus, I worked for several offices as a salaried employee, mostly as a general practitioner, and tried to open my own practice. Finally Dr. Samuel Bolonik, an American-born and trained pediatrician, was looking for a successor to his practice in suburban Chicago, a practice he had built over more than forty years, and he took me on as his junior partner.

Though I had been practicing in the United States for two years at this time, I consider that my real American pediatric experience began in 1980, when I joined Dr. Bolonik's office. There I found myself, as I had in the Soviet Union, working exclusively with children—a job that I feel I can do better than any other.

One of my greatest challenges was communication. My Russian accent was at that time even more pronounced, and I had little knowledge of how to speak on the same wavelength as my patients and their parents or of how to erase the cultural barrier between my patients' families and me.

Dr. Bolonik retired two years later, but working with him for those two years was an invaluable and irreplaceable experience for me.

Dr. Bolonik, who was a pediatric legend in his community, opened the door to American practice for me and was an important model of professional behavior.

I soon learned that there was not that much difference between Russian and American patients; the main difference was the parents. To discuss the difference between Russian and American parents would take a book in itself, but for all their superficial differences, the basic psychology is the same: parents on both sides of the ocean love their children and passionately want health, peace, and happiness for them.

Looking back on my early relationships with my American patients, I see that at first, I did not understand the many nuances of the American character. For me the main feature of this character is behavior, which is typical for people who grew up in political freedom, people who can express themselves well and are not ashamed to be themselves. My growing understanding of American psychology and, probably, the reputation that I have established for more than fifteen years have made my contacts with my patients and their families much easier and more natural. Despite my experience, however, I still encounter cases where I reach my limit of understanding with my interlocutors, and they do not understand me at all.

Nevertheless, based on my experience, I believe that when people are truly concerned, they can come close to understanding each other. The truly necessary ingredient is the goodwill of both parties involved in the dialogue.

THE SILENT VISITORS

For a long time, one of my most challenging tasks was dealing with "silent parents." These parents bring their children to the office for a visit but then like to pretend they are not there, avoid speaking to the pediatrician, and challenge the pediatrician to come up with a diagnosis without any knowledge of the history of the condition that brought the child to the office in the first place. Though silent parents are all somehow intimidating, they can be divided into three different categories: the first group is genuinely trying to intimidate the physician, the second group is only tired, and the third group is habitually withdrawn.

The body language of intimidating parents frequently expresses their unverbalized resentment. Their unspoken message often is, "Guess what *I* am thinking now. After your guesses you might hear something from me that will really surprise you." The tired group usually consists of parents who are bringing their children for an office visit after working the night shift. The withdrawn parents have something on their mind that diverts them from the reason for their visit to the pediatrician's office.

I learned about these different types from life; nobody teaches this in medical school or in pediatric residencies. Until I learned about these different types of silent parents and their behaviors, their visits were very stressful and demanding. Life became much easier for me once I accumulated enough experience of working with these people. To deal with these parents, I have developed the "Gorbachev method," wherein in order to alleviate the situation I use *glasnost* (openness) to communicate with the parents. Though this method did not work well for Gorbachev, it has worked fairly well for me over the past several years and has saved me from much unnecessary adrenaline production and peptic ulcers.

It is better to talk things over, even if what I hear from a parent is very unpleasant, than to be in a state of anxious expectation and uncertainty during, and sometimes even after, the visit.

Since this discovery I have been surprised to realize that the vast majority of parents do not have anything against their child's pediatrician; rather, they bring their unresolved conflicts and bad associations to the office along with their children. With all types of silent parents, but especially with parents of the tired or the withdrawn type, the Gorbachev method immediately resolves a tense situation that, only moments before, looked like a big problem.

April Price, a four-year-old, was brought to my office by her grandmother, Mrs. Black, who was a registered nurse at a nearby hospital. April's symptoms were increased frequency of urination and pain in her lower abdomen. The most likely cause was a urinary tract infection. While I was examining my patient and waiting for the results of her urinalysis to come back, April's grandmother did not once open her mouth on her own initiative.

In a urinary tract infection, the history of the illness has a decisive importance for establishment of a diagnosis. My patient had been treated with home remedies by her grandmother before coming to me, and this made obtaining information even more important. Having no other alternative, I repeatedly tried to obtain more information from Mrs. Black, who sat in my office with an apathetic and withdrawn look on her face.

Not having received any meaningful information from Mrs. Black after a substantial amount of time, I took a deep breath and remarked, "I see there is something that's bothering you, Mrs. Black. Let's get it out in the open. Tell me why you are so silent."

I could see Mrs. Black beginning to surface and the light of consciousness beginning to show in her face. I realized that I might become the object of her anger once she started talking, but I could no longer stand this blank look and her lack of cooperation.

"I mean that I see a lot of tension in your face and would like to help both of us to find a solution," I continued.

Finally, I saw that Mrs. Black was ready to become fully awake, like Sleeping Beauty after the kiss from the loving prince.

She looked at me. Thought. Thought again. Blew her nose. I then saw an apologetic smile on her absorbed face.

"Oh, it's nothing, Doctor. Pardon me. I had surgery on my right wrist three days ago, and it's still bothering me, though I took some Tylenol with codeine twice today. It's nothing against you."

A few years ago I was examining a fourteen-year-old boy for abdominal pain. He was accompanied by his attractive, middle-aged mother. From the moment I entered the room, I saw that Mrs. Jankowski was tense, distracted, and uncommunicative. After going through much speculation, I could not arrive at any reason for her nervousness. After a quarter of an hour she still remained silent, had not uttered more than one or two phases, and still avoided looking at me.

Enough is enough, I said to myself. "Mrs. Jankowski, is something wrong? Did I do something to cause you to practically refuse to speak to me?"

Mrs. Jankowski looked at me as if I had awakened her from a bad dream.

"Oh, Doctor," she answered softly in a sad voice, "I am so sorry. It's nothing to do with you. My uncle was killed in a car accident two days ago. Don't pay any attention to me. I'll be all right."

BITTERSWEET VICTORIES

NOT ALL of the beneficial changes that physicians can achieve in their office for the short office visit are victories in the long run. After a fleeting moment that affects a child's personality positively comes the realization that the bright moment of success is inevitably fated to be dissolved by the uncompromising realities of life.

"Doctor, you'd better go to room four before you see the next patient. Clara Rodale is out of control in there. She has been crying, yelling, shaking, and drooling in there for more than fifteen minutes. Please don't delay."

Svetlana, my medical assistant, presented me with this challenge, and I was not sure whether I would be able to withstand it. Feeling like a trainer entering a cage containing a wild animal, I entered the examining room.

My "animal" was only six years old and at the peak of a temper tantrum. I could hear all kinds of incongruous sounds, punctuated with spitting, screaming, and swearing. This commotion was coming from under a desk, where I usually sit in the examining room. There, on the floor in the far corner I saw Clara Rodale lying in a fetal position.

I had not seen Clara in my office before—she was not a new patient, but she had been examined by the other pediatricians in the office on her three prior visits, though she had never been such a behavioral disaster as today. While Clara persisted in her wild emotional outburst, I asked her mother, Lynn Morgan, many questions about her daughter. In her late thirties, Lynn had the face of a woman, who in the course of life's tribulations, had detached herself from her feelings. Lynn sat very straight in her chair as if she had swallowed a stick and answered my questions mechanically, in a robotlike manner. It was obvious that she had been through these tantrums numerous times in many different places.

Even to an inexperienced observer it was clear that Clara had a serious emotional problem. This problem, as I later learned had caused her school system to place her in a special class for children with behavioral problems. She had not done well in this class either. With the dispassionate appearance of a person who was resigned to her destiny, Lynn told me, to an accompaniment of yelling, screaming, and crying produced by her daughter, the abridged story of her family.

She had been divorced from Clara's father two years earlier. Clara's father now saw his daughter only once a month. The last time he saw Clara, he presented her with a present—a small kitten, the care of which was automatically assumed by Lynn and her new husband, whom she had married ten months before. Her new marriage did not appear to be an example of a happy marital union, either. The last two months she and her new husband had been working different shifts at their jobs and had barely seen each other. With the tired appearance of a resolute martyr, Lynn told me that she felt sure that her new husband was intentionally trying to minimize his contact with his difficult stepdaughter.

After this conversation I switched my attention to Clara. I addressed her in a normal and natural manner, trying to transmit to her the unspoken message that though I noticed her reaction and took it for what it was, I also knew other, more appropriate ways of controlling the situation that would work better than her tantrums and that I would be happy to share my knowledge with her. I had hoped to let Clara know in a friendly, yet at the same time firm and consistent manner, that I took her reaction as an immature conduct that she subconsciously used out of a desire to retain her infantile omnipotence and to escape from the reality of having to follow somebody's orders. At the same time I wanted to convey to her my regret at the opportunities she missed by clinging to her improper, babyish behavior. If she responded, I would then give her some hints as to how to behave in complicated situations in a more grown-up way, thus helping her to avoid her chosen destructive demeanor.

In different circumstances, I was similarly helped once during my own childhood. When I was ten years old, I ran through a wide, dark, school corridor at a late evening hour when there were not many students around. I slipped on the wet linoleum floor and fell down. Though I was in pain, it would not have prevented me from pulling myself up and continuing on my way, but at this moment I heard the voice of Pyotr Dmitrievich Illyichev, the physics teacher who was our school favorite.

I assumed the position of an injured victim, hardly breathing, as if I was about to pass out. In a moment I had regressed at least eight years and was subconsciously anticipating from my teacher the reaction of an anxious parent who sees his or her child in distress. He walked with older children toward the place where I lay like a wounded hero, and as he reached me, he leaned over, carefully looked at my face, and touched my legs and hands. Then, with a note of an unforgettable subdued irony, but without a trace of contempt for my transformation to a baby, he stroked my hair and in a caring voice, ignoring the fact that I was lying motionless on the floor with my eyes closed, said to me, "OK, Vladimir, you are in good shape. You can now stand up and go where you were planning to go. Go."

He then left me and walked away with his group. I quickly stood up and limped away as fast as I could. In an instant I was cured from a self-induced syncopal episode and never resorted to it again.

Now, many years later, I was trying to communicate with my young patient in the same manner during her tantrum. To my satisfaction I noticed that the more I talked to Clara, the less she pretended that she could not hear me. Finally, her head and then the rest of her came out from her under-desk asylum.

Now was the time to use another powerful mechanism of intervention—the indispensable tool of distraction. Minutes later we were flying like two birds all over the office. In each room we entered I showed Clara different toys, flashing contraptions, and colored lights. Soon, we went back to her mother with Clara jumping and laughing.

Svetlana was standing in the doorway looking at us when we, like two friends, returned to the examining room. She was amazed to witness the startling change in Clara.

On seeing the reaction of Clara's mother, however, I could not fully share Svetlana's enthusiasm. Instead of showing pleased surprise to her daughter's transformation to a merry girl, Lynn's appearance expressed her pessimism about this metamorphosis. She obviously felt that the change in her daughter's conduct would not be long-lived; Lynn was anticipating her reversion back to "a spoiled brat" and had no belief that her own behavior could affect Clara's just as mine had. She had cast herself as a victim and martyr who took all the burden of Clara's care, while I was just someone who was trying to impress her with smoke-and-mirrors sophisticated tricks and would forget about this patient, her daughter, as soon as they left the office.

My hope that Clara might have a good chance for psychological improvement was reduced by the realization that she had been inexorably caught up in her mother's psychological problem—it was clear to me that Lynn had chosen the role of martyr and did not want to change her own self-destructive, masochistic tendencies.

My attempts to discuss my observations with Lynn were met with impervious resistance. Dedicated to suffering, she defended her neurosis like an intrepid warrior who fought for sacred spiritual values. There are laws against the physical abuse of children, but there are no laws—nor would their enforcement be possible if such laws existed—concerning parents who are detrimentally affecting their child's mind in a much more subtle psychological manner. If, for example, Lynn were beating her daughter, intervention would be possible and could be effective, but this much more dangerous and pernicious influence on the child's developing personality was out of realm of intervention unless Lynn herself decided that she needed to be helped.

So it was destined: Clara will continue to study in the special class, and her mother will probably divorce her second husband and silently, without complaint, suffer the rest of her life, refusing to understand that she and her daughter, whom she without a doubt loves in her own manner, might be helped.

But.... miracles happen. All the time.

TRIP TO ARIZONA

ONCE, A long time ago, I thought that my goodwill could transform and win out against any situation if I tried my hardest. The older I get, the more I realize the limitations to my intervention. In cases where I feel that I cannot do anything constructive for a family, I try to relax and just listen.

The call I received from Mrs. Simer caught me at a good time. It was the slow season—approximately between the beginning of June and the first three weeks of July—when children are not usually sick and need no school physical. The availability of my time allowed me to answer all of Mrs. Simer's questions to the best of my ability instead of politely letting her know that she was asking questions that she ought to try to solve by herself.

Mrs. Simer had just recently become a mother for the first time. Her newborn child, a boy, was at the time of this conversation only six weeks old. Mrs. Simer had accumulated several questions that she had tried to solve with her husband and girlfriends. Unable to find any good solutions, she had, on the advice of her girlfriends, who were no doubt exasperated with her, decided to contact her pediatrician, me. I expressed my appreciation to Mrs. Simer on being told how I had been selected for such a responsible role.

We began our telephone chat with a discussion on some different aspects of a trip to Arizona the family was planning. In a solemn and proud tone Mrs. Simer told me that she and her husband would be traveling to the state of Arizona in four months time. In light of this trip she began asking me what I thought about hot weather. She told me that she did not like hot weather, and she had already made this point to her husband in a most determined manner.

Listening to the intensity and passion in Mrs. Simer voice, I surmised that she was not looking for medical advice but was instead trying, with my help, to prove her point in a marital conflict. That still did not prevent me from expressing my professional opinion. "Hot or cold," I said, "it is not prudent to travel for very long distances in a car with a small baby."

"Okay," responded Mrs. Simer, who was satisfied with this answer. "Then I have another question for you. Suppose my husband wins, and we decide to go on this vacation, anyway. In that case, what will happen with the breast-feeding of my baby?"

"Why should anything happen with your baby's breast-feeding, Mrs. Simer?"

"Would it not present a danger to my baby?"

"Mrs. Simer," I protested, "breast-feeding, as a general rule, presents a great advantage for babies. Breast is best!"

"Doctor," my interlocutress objected in a dignified tone, "to breast-feed my baby I would need to unfasten his car seat to bring it and the baby close to my breast. This will not only present an inconvenience for the baby in getting to my breast but could also present a serious danger if something happened to the car during the time I was feeding him."

"But, Mrs. Simer," I said, grateful that this conversation was happening now—it was obvious that Mrs. Simer, endowed with plenty of free time, was actively fighting boredom and could have called me about these issues after midnight—"did you ever think that you might feed your baby while the car is parked? Then, not only would your baby's safety be ensured, but, also, you would not need to unfasten the car seat with the baby in it. Instead of schlepping a child and a car seat combination, you could simply pick up the child!"

"You see, Doctor, I knew we were going to come to a good decision," the young mother said, praising me for my efforts to help her. "But I still think there could be a better solution to my problem."

I expressed my regret that I could not be of more help.
"Now to go on to my next question," announced Mrs. Simer. "What do you think about my painting the inside of my house?"

"Though I am not a painter, I don't see any reason that you shouldn't decorate your house."

"But, Doctor, there is the baby in the house."

"Why didn't you fix up your house before the baby was born?" I asked the young mother as I tried to hide my annoyance.

"You know, that is exactly what I ask myself when I see the mess my house is in now. But I have another question regarding the trip to *Arizonia*. Suppose I do not breast feed the baby and he is on formula instead. Suppose. How many four-ounce bottles or twelve ounce cans should I take with us if we are planning to travel for about eight hours a day for four days without stopping for gas?"

I was never good with arithmetic so I asked Mrs. Simer to hold this question for the next four months until she was ready to depart on her trip. I had to return to my office schedule, and I explained this to her. Because Mrs. Simer was upset that she could not ask me more questions, I decided to entertain her. "With these enormous travel-related problems you have," I joked, "you might feel that the trip is not worth all the worries. You stay at home, and I will go instead of you. Ok?"

"Doctor," Mrs. Simer said with injured dignity, "if I decide not to go, then my husband will not go either. We do not travel separately."

I understood that I should look for another way to get my vacation.

GOOD DOCTORS, BAD DOCTORS

"ALL THE world's a stage, and all the men and women merely players." Like anyone else, I am not immune to playing a role that, sometimes with the best intentions but against my desire, is imposed on me. With Mrs. Beverly Mackin, a woman with a bubbling, happy personality, I played a game called "Good Doctors, Bad Doctors."

Her daughter, Barbara, had become a patient in my office about six months prior to this follow-up visit. Mrs. Mackin found our office listed in the booklet given to her by her insurance company, not by word of mouth as was usually the case until the managed health care era.

The two most remarkable features about Mrs. Mackin were her large ball-like body and her open, delightful face. Her face had been adorned by nature with large, animated, brown eyes and a youthful, sincere smile.

She worked as a clerk and was happily married. Her marriage may have taken place in her relatively mature years as Barbara was only eight years old at this time, and Mrs. Mackin was thirty eight. Barbara was, overall, a very normal child; her only problem was that she was too active, or hyperactive, and this interfered with her school activities. The syndrome that makes children to be unable to concentrate on educational tasks because of their hyperactivity is called attention deficit disorder. Paradoxically, in order for Barbara to concentrate on her schoolwork better, she needed to take a medication called Ritalin® which stimulates the nervous system. The best explanation for this paradox that I could find in medical literature was that though a child is very active and, therefore, appears to be alert, the child is still unable to concentrate on intellectual tasks. A stimulant helps children with this disorder "wake up" to abstract thinking, thus creating a condition where the learning process can be brought to the focus of attention.

When I left the USSR nothing was known there about using stimulants for hyperactive children, and my initial attitude about using them in the treatment of hyperactivity was extremely cautious. My common sense could not accept the possibility that a "pep" pill that would create a brainstorm in a normal, healthy individual who took it might produce the opposite effect when taken by a hyperactive child. Nevertheless, to my complete surprise, numerous children and their parents and teachers confirmed the helpful effects of this drug, and this eventually persuaded me that for some children with hyperactivity this medication is definitely beneficial. Whenever I prescribe this medication, I follow the patient very closely, especially during the first month or two of treatment, to make sure that the medicine is working and is not producing any side effects.

When Barbara became my patient, she was already taking Ritalin®, and our first visit was dedicated to obtaining a careful history of her condition. Barbara's previous pediatrician, Dr. Nelson, either did not believe in the curative action of Ritalin® or was very worried about its side effects. He made Mrs. Mackin very nervous whenever she went in with her daughter for a visit and a Ritalin® refill. The memories about these encounters made Mrs. Mackin very tense during Barbara's first visit to me, but as soon as she saw that her feeling that Ritalin® was helping her child was fully trusted, she became relaxed, friendly, and talkative. Though she was a very busy working mother, I was able to persuade her that periodic reevaluations in the office were necessary as long as her superhealthy daughter was taking such a strong drug.

One of my greatest "friends" in the office is the sound system, which allows me to listen to my favorite music. Though I might be in working, and the span of my life seems to be decreasing exactly proportionally to the time spent in the office, music allows me to exist in a dimension beyond my job without causing the quality of my work to suffer. During some difficult times when the appropriate decision was critical to a child's recovery, the familiar sounds of my favorite music reassuringly provided me with the emotional support I needed to find the best solution for the situation.

My office musical repertoire consists mostly of classical music, but on this day we were listening to Italian folk songs in the office. Somewhere on the subconscious level the familiar melodies that were known to me from childhood were warming my heart and filling me with a sense of well-being as I examined my patient.

Before I could sit at my desk to write a note in Barbara's record and her prescription, I heard Mrs. Mackin's high, melodious voice. "Why do you like Italian music? Are you an Italian?" she asked, looking straight at me.

"No," I replied, "I am not an Italian, but I was born and lived in Europe."

The strains of one of my favorite songs "O, Sole Mio," which was playing then, connected my presence in the office at that moment with my past life experience, and I added, "Like you, I am a citizen of this planet called Earth, and I like to find in every nation of the world all that is lovely and beautiful."

Beverly looked at me with great interest.

"You know, I feel the same way as you," she said slowly, and then, in a singing and impassioned voice she added, "and I adore you, Doctor!"

Though I know how fickle human vanity is, still, it was pleasant for me to hear these words of praise. Not only were they as dear to me as a present, but I also feel I need them in some way as a mathematical unit, as a sort of "credit" against all the negative events that occur in my professional life. If—as is inevitable for me as a person who works directly with other people—someone should give a negative evaluation of me as a physician or as a person, I can balance this debit against the credit of Beverly's praise and can come to a spiritual contentment. This is one of many ways to achieve a state that might be called a professional nirvana.

In appreciation of our mutual understanding and friendship, Beverly and I hugged each other, and I then proceeded to fill out the necessary paperwork to conclude the visit.

"I feel very comfortable in your office," Beverly said as I wrote "I'm so glad I changed doctors. With my previous Dr. Nelson, I never had such a good time."

It is difficult to discern what is objective and what is subjective when a patient who has changed doctors complains about the previous medical office. Though I usually try to avoid such conversations, as they are a waste of time and can frequently become quite emotional, it would have been rude to interrupt Beverly, and I thought that she perhaps needed to vent her feelings about the previous doctor.

She was criticizing Dr. Nelson, whom I did not know very well, for his sloppiness and poor bedside manners, but for some reason the main cause of her disapproval was Dr. Nelson's hair.

Indeed, his thick black hair did sometimes stick out from his head and later, once he began to grow a beard, it was unruly as well. For Mrs. Mackin, Dr. Nelson's hair was an impediment to the provision of medical care to her daughter. If I was to take seriously what Beverly was saying, I would have been led to believe that Dr. Nelson specially kept his hair in its chaotic disarray just to irritate Mrs. Mackin and, additionally, to intimidate her daughter, who had enough psychological problems without being affected by his pediatrician's hair.

While I listened to Beverly, it occurred to me that though she might be trying to be objective in her assessment of the previous pediatrician and his hair, someone else might find Dr. Nelson's wild black hair to be a thing of natural beauty and originality.

I only hoped that if the parents who once used my services ever start taking their children to Dr. Nelson's office and criticize me for my, at times, unruly gray hair, Dr. Nelson would try to be as philosophical as I was trying to be when someone disapproved of him in my presence.

Finally, Barbara received the traditional little present at the end of the visit, and Beverly and I went through our last round of expressing our mutual trust, admiration, and happiness in seeing one another. We parted as two old friends, each of us faithfully performing our part in the wonderful play called life.

A SATISFIED PARENT

COMMUNICATION BETWEEN people creates the bridge that allows them to coexist.

From the minute I began my conversation with Cynthia Bartlett, I felt that I had to concentrate on each word she said to understand exactly what she meant by her disorganized speech.

Mrs. Bartlett was not satisfied with the explanations given by previous doctors about her daughter's condition. She had brought her eighteen-month-old child, Nicole, not for a second, but for a third doctor's opinion on the child's peculiar medical condition—a condition that had made Mrs. Bartlett quite nervous and upset. A battery of laboratory tests that had previously been done didn't elicit any abnormalities on Nicole.

It did not take a long time to understand what stood in the way of establishing a diagnosis. Cynthia was a disaster from the standpoint of communication: she talked with an emotional excitement and anxiety that—or so at least it seemed to me—she wanted to pass on to me as well. This hysteria was further enhanced by her mannerisms and her piercing and unwavering, mesmerizing stare.

In a short time I learned that I could not match Cynthia's hypnotizing ability, and I stopped trying to "outlook" her unblinking gaze. The only way out of the spell of Mrs. Bartlett's was to listen to her while looking at her daughter. That, however, would mean that I had capitulated to her subconscious urge to control me, her partner in conversation. I chose a much more effective way: though I kept looking in the direction of Cynthia's eyes, I focused behind her head and stared straight into infinity.

Mrs. Bartlett's manner betrayed not her emotional strength, but her emotional weakness. With her intimidating, pseudoaggressive appearance, she was trying to cover her insecurities and her inability to communicate in a mature, give-and-take manner.

The reflexive and unprofessional way to react to such an attitude is to answer it in mirror fashion: excitement for excitement, scream for scream. Eventually, this is the road to conflict. Besides, Mrs. Bartlett, whose daughter's health was providing her with a golden alibi, would immediately use this lack of respect toward her as an indication of a lack of sensitivity to her daughter's problem.

A more professional way to deal with this kind of situation is to listen carefully to what such parents are saying, try to accumulate the necessary information, asking questions, if possible, and then at an appropriate moment, approach the parents in such a way that they will turn their speech from an abstract, detached, and amorphous form to a concrete presentation of facts.

After silently listening to Mrs. Bartlett's monologue for a good amount of time, during which I was looking at Cynthia with a tragically serious face, I stood up, approached Mrs. Bartlett, and took her hand in my hand while she continued her incessant talking. Then, giving as friendly a smile as I could—no, it was not the insincere smile of a politician because I was doing what was in the best interest of my patient and because I could well predict Cynthia's reaction—I said to her with affection, "Boy, you have such a beautiful little girl. Nicole is dressed like a little princess. Tell me, where do you buy her clothing?"

Mrs. Bartlett looked at me, first dubiously, but then smiled and proudly told me that she had bought Nicole's outfit at Madigans. It was bought especially for this visit.

After this and a couple of other relaxing, conversational questions, our talk became more organized and systematic: Mrs. Bartlett had received a polite and unspoken message that she was not in control of the situation. Previous experience had taught me that with this turn of the tables there was a good chance not only that Cynthia would begin answering my questions to the point but that she might even allow me to give my opinion about different aspects of Nicole's condition.

This did, in fact, happen: Cynthia straightaway allowed our talk to become a conversation instead of a monologue, and, little by little, I started to grasp her daughter's problem. The reason it had initially been so difficult to understand the main complaint was that previously Mrs. Bartlett had been trying to emphasize that her daughter's problem was with her bowel movements. Whenever I asked whether it was diarrhea or constipation that was the problem, however, Cynthia denied that it was either.

Finally, Mrs. Bartlett was able to explain her observations: whenever little Nicole used the bathroom "for #2," which usually happened once a day, she tried to hide herself, but when her mother observed her inconspicuously, she saw that Nicole was rubbing her legs and rocking from side to side with her eyes closed until her face would turn red and that she would begin to perspire, and her body would shake.

"Why," Cynthia exclaimed, as I thought about my answer, "why is she reacting in this way!"

The diagnosis of Nicole's condition was simple: she had discovered masturbation as a pleasurable experience. But would Mrs. Bartlett accept this diagnosis without responding to it in a hysterical fashion?

Waiting for some kind of reaction from Cynthia, I explained sentence by sentence what, in my opinion, her daughter had and told her that she should try to ignore Nicole's activity as long as she did not do it in public or excessively. "It's a variant of normal sexuality," I said in conclusion, keeping in mind the young age of my patient. "Relax and let her do it."

Surprisingly, Mrs. Bartlett, who was now attentively listening to me while she chewed in a rhythmic manner on a large piece of gum, accepted my diagnosis with satisfaction and gratitude.

"You know," she told me, "I could not, kind of, well, explain it to you very clearly, but epilepsy runs in my family so I was worried that Nicole was having seizures each time she pooped. Now I understand it."

There were no more questions, and Mrs. Bartlett left the office visibly satisfied.

A month later I heard a loud female voice in one of the examining rooms. On entering, I saw Cynthia and her daughter. This time Nicole had been brought in for a well-baby visit.

"How about her earlier problem?" I inquired of Cynthia.

"What problem? Oh, that! No problem. We are doing OK with that."

I did not try to clarify exactly what she meant by "that."

UNIVERSAL VALUES

PHYSICIAN-PARENT or, in the case of a pediatrician, physician-family relations are, in these times of managed and third-party regulated care, becoming progressively more bureaucratized, with the introduction of many barriers between both parties.

Nobody said it better than my beautiful five-year-old patient Leah Panich. After watching me diligently write in her chart a voluminous note in order to satisfy the requirements of CPT—current procedure terminology—coding, requirements that are closely watched by clerks from different insurance companies and by lawyers who specialize in doctor intimidation, she asked her mother what I was doing.

"Don't you see," her mother answered. "He is writing a note about your problem."

Leah, who was not yet educated in the modern health industry trends, said to her mother with reproach, "I don't understand this. Doctors should not write about people. They should speak with children and treat them. To write is for writers, for doctors—to check and to treat."

One outcome of the new health care trend is the feeling of suspicion on the part of the family that the primary doctor's loyalties are split between the patient and the insurance company or managed care organization. This suspicion is the result of the influence of the news media, of the family's friends, and, sometimes, of the family's own experience. Frequently, patients, instead of seeing their doctor in the friendly way that is portrayed in old-time books and movies, see a person who has a physician's license but who, as far as their insurance company is concerned, is a "gatekeeper" in the "cafeteria" of available health care services. Patients do not see the physician as a member of their extended family; they see him or her only as a person who has the responsibility of providing for the technical needs of their health.

For example, as a part of the contractual relationship with a managed care organization, a physician is responsible for keeping a patient from seeing specialists as long as the physician feels that the patient's case can be managed in the office; the physician is discouraged from ordering unnecessary, expensive tests. Medicine, however, is an art and not only a science, and sometimes the opinions of the physician and the patient may differ, causing some patients to harbor the suspicion that they are being deprived of top-quality health care.

Though an unsophisticated patient who has no chronic health condition requiring special treatment may not know the specifics of the physician-family relationship in a managed care organization setting, my new patient, Mrs. Singh, knew it well. She was a medical technologist who had recently transferred to my practice from another pediatrician who also participated in this managed care organization; she transferred because of some conflict whose details I did not know. Looking at her, I saw that she already did not trust me. She had done her homework to prepare herself for obtaining from me, as the primary physician, all that she felt was necessary for her child's health care, and she was ready to fight me for it.

Mrs. Singh was the mother of a special child. Her six-year-old son, Navin, whose handsome face retained the features of his Indian descent, also carried the universal features of a condition that mercilessly afflicts children of all races. Navin's eyes had epicanthic folds, and he had a large tongue and a short, fleshy neck. It was obvious that this child had Down's syndrome, a genetic condition in which one of the chromosomes, chromosome 21, is abnormally translocated. (In translocation, a part of the chromosome is detached from its normal position and is attached to another chromosome).

Down's syndrome occurs in every racial group, regardless of how superior this group might think itself; it equalizes all human beings by causing those born with the condition to look like twins, whether they are born to European, African, or Asian parents.

Though the appearance of the little good-natured boy clearly showed Down's syndrome, it was for me a pity to realize that he suffered from this congenital condition, which affects the mental abilities, motor abilities, and internal organs of the children who have it, and thus I tried to deny my impression and to think of something less dramatic to explain the appearance of my visitor. In searching for help in this vain attempt, I turned towards Navin's mother, who stood beside her son, and gently asked an open question. "Does he have?" I asked her as I looked straight into her eyes.

"Yes, he has Down's syndrome." Mrs. Singh finished my question and turned her eyes immediately to her son's face, looking at him with a concentrated gaze. I wanted to continue our conversation and tried to ask a few more questions, but Mrs. Singh was not willing to talk and answered me as she would any person who was collecting information only for the sake of bureaucratic reasons and not out of genuine human interest.

Being the mother of a Down's syndrome child—or of any child with a visible congenital defect—presents a challenge in itself, and so it was natural that she would not want to open her heart to a pediatrician who, according to her health management organization HMO's booklet, was not even called a physician or a doctor but PCP, "a primary care provider." I anticipated her hesitation and, from experience, assumed that she did not expect much from me or from the visit to my office.

As I tried to obtain more information about her child's past history to become better acquainted with the family and with the child, Mrs. Singh deflected my questions with a manner that lacked all enthusiasm. All she wanted on this day was to get a prescription for Navin's cold and to get a referral to a dermatologist. She saw me as a person who took down information for irrelevant but official bureaucratic purposes.

Though we belonged to the same species and were located less than a foot apart, Mrs. Singh seemed to exist in a different world; she had come to me only and exclusively for the problems she had already told me about, so why mess around with all this conversation? It was written all over her face: Give me my prescription, give me my referral, and let me go. There is nothing to talk about. We are strangers.

Though Mrs. Singh was entitled to her opinion, I was not ready to share her skeptical outlook on my function as a doctor. While it is true that the label "PCP" that I carried, thanks to the managed care organization's new age semantics, equalized me with all people in the medical profession and was taking away my professional identity, I still considered myself a doctor, and to me that means that I ought to offer my patients more than just prescriptions and referrals.

It was not Mrs. Singh's fault that she perceived my profession in the way that the managed health care industry wanted her to; she understood literally what the other party wanted her to believe. Against my will, I felt that it was my moral obligation to prove her wrong. I continued our conversation in order to ask a series of questions, to which I received curt answers from Mrs. Singh, until I obtained the necessary information on Navin's past health history. I then paused.

While Mrs. Singh hurriedly dressed her son, I approached Navin and stroked his head.

"Your son," I said, "though he has Down's syndrome, is, luckily, not profoundly affected by this condition. Anyone can see that he is very handsome and intelligent. Recently I read in a journal a piece of poetry that had been written by an Israeli girl who had Down's syndrome. I am positive that Navin will be able to be a good student, and, one fine day, he will be able to hold a job and earn his own money." I spoke solely for the sake of my own conscience, not expecting very much from this woman I had only just met. Thus, it was completely unexpected when I noticed the unmistakable signs of Mrs. Singh's lively interest in what I was saying.

Her dark eyes, which had been lifeless only a moment before, suddenly became filled with curiosity and natural intelligence. I could see that she was catching each word I said, and, seeing her genuine interest, I took a deep breath and told her that I felt really sorry that her son had been born with this condition and that she, as a mother, had to deal with it. "But," I told her, "you are a great mother; otherwise God would not give him to you. He gave him to you and to your husband because He knew that you had enough strength to raise him and to love him the way you do."

It was not the first time in my long pediatric career that I was able to establish contact with a parent, but the miraculous, dramatic outcome of our conversation is impossible to forget. The ice melted between us. The differences in our upbringing—our race, age, gender, and social position—were no longer of any import. We became a part of the same world, "the planet of people," as the French author Antoine de Saint-Exupéry called it in one of his famous books.

We shook hands cordially at the end of the conversation. As I left the examining room, I thought that in our century of "isms" and of numerous attempts by all kinds of self-proclaimed and elected-by-no-one activists to categorize people into an infinite number of groups based on the different races, religions, nationalities, genders, languages, and even street addresses, mankind would be able to save many millions of human lives if we began judging "others" not on the basis of what separates us, and makes us different, but on the solid and fundamental things that unite us, that are universal to us.

For Mrs. Singh and me this solid and fundamental thing was our human compassion—the caring and warmth of human beings.

4

LISTENING TO CHILDREN

Since becoming a pediatrician in 1964, I have been surrounded by the talk of children nearly every day. Initially, I thought hearing their talk was just fun, but as I gained more experience, I began to understand that I could learn plenty by listening to children and that some of their talk might be of great help to me in my practice. Listening to children not only allows me to appreciate their development but also gives me an opportunity to peek at their souls and become acquainted with their unique personalities.

Each time I see a newborn, I have the opportunity to observe an unsurpassed miracle. Only months before, this human being did not exist but was just becoming; then suddenly an individual endowed with a first and last name enters into the world, which is, as yet, unknown to him or her. A child's development is like walking down a road trying different paths: by trial and error the developing youngster learns the relationship between cause and effect.

Children's language, which to many people seems funny and senseless, is actually a long journey into the world of adults. By listening to their speech, we can perceive the reflection of our own development in its evolution to mature consciousness. Their speech reflects the world they see, which they describe in a sincere and open manner because they have not yet learned how to conceal their thoughts.

TIME FLIES

FEDELE VERNI, a long-standing patient of mine who was six, was brought, along with his older sister, Victoria, to my office by his grandfather. Victoria was suffering from a slight respiratory illness. Their mother was unable to bring them, as she was working as a clerk in a store; a job she began when her husband, Andrew, divorced her the year before. Andrew now finds himself in the situation of many men his age: he began a new family and now uses my services for the child born of his second marriage. I wait for the day when, by an accident of scheduling, his old and new families cross paths in my office.

Fedele and Victoria both feel quite comfortable in my office, as they have come here since they were newborns. Fedele, in fact, pretty much acts as if he owns the place. As always, he was taking a very active role in each detail of conversation. For some reason I was asking what Victoria's age was. "Ten," she replied.

"Ten!" exclaimed Fedele, incredulous at such an advanced age. When his sister confirmed her age, I saw an expression on Fedele's face that, were he an adult, would be called philosophical. "I thought you were eight!"

Unable to hide his sincere amazement, he stared at Victoria and was lost in his private musing. Thus, I was present at the moment when, at an early age, Fedele discovered the meaning of the expression "Time fleeth away without delay."

I looked over to Fedele's grandfather, and we each gave a knowing smile.

TO NEW HORIZONS

THE DAGGETT family is an example of a genuinely intact nuclear family. For more than the last decade the family's bread and butter has been provided by the state's welfare system. Nina Daggett, whom I met twelve years ago, was a small woman, barely into her thirties with sparkling eyes, and a wide, disarming smile on her amiable face. She has always been a housewife, while her husband, Marcus, has worked at a variety of jobs over the years. Five years ago, for instance, he though he might have a vocation for the ministry and tried that for a time. During this period he came into my office looking very dignified in a black shirt and a religious collar. He was very natural as a man of the cloth, and though his career as a minister did not last very long, from then on he wore a solemn and dignified expression on his full bearded face that, together with his natural intelligence and excellent sense of humor, made each meeting with him a delight.

Though Marcus had never worked on a regular basis, he was an outstanding parent, as was his wife, and, together, they had brought up their children with the best possible care. Their entire lives were devoted to rearing their offspring. Even though Marcus and Nina were legally married, they were able to remain on the welfare rolls, maybe, among other reasons, because the social workers at the department of public aid were so impressed with their genuine parental involvement with their children.

Having been their pediatrician since their first child was born, I felt happy that their children, unlike so many others in my practice, had both parents available for nurture and support.

Though the Daggett children were active and noisy when they came to my office, they were also respectful of adults and easy to reason with. All six of the children (including a set of twins) were under twelve years of age.

Two years ago one of the more aggressive managed care organizations that were looking for new patients among welfare recipients had deftly coerced the Daggetts into joining its group. This HMO underestimated the intelligence of the Daggetts. Not only were the Daggetts released from the HMO's roster and placed back under my services, but, to our common satisfaction, the HMO apologized for its piratical methods of business practice.

When the twins Eddie and Andrew were two years old, they came into my office for a follow-up exam after having had chickenpox. With the marks of that infection still upon them, they were sitting next to each other on the examining table energetically talking and laughing.

As I examined them, Nina shared her amazement over the twins' developmental progress with her husband and me. She then told me how much her children like to come to my office and how at home they feel here. I declared my similar feelings for her family and then, trying to keep the conversation going, expressed my regret that Andrew, who was such a big boy, was still not fully toilet trained. His parents had decided to try potty-training the twins—Eddie and Andrew were trusted to go out without their diapers—and the large damp patch on Andrew's clean pants betrayed his still-poor control over his bladder. His brother's pants, however, were dry; so far he had met his parents' expectations.

Nina, with the happiest and kindest smile in the world, reproached her number 2 twin with, "Andrew, baby, why did you pee in your pants? Aren't you a big boy?"

Her beloved son gave her an unforgettable look, which expressed both immaculate innocence and his strong belief that he was to be exempted from boring and not-of-his-age-interest responsibilities. Blinding his mother with his own sunshine smile, he bent his right arm and, pointing with his left index finger to his powerful two-year-old's biceps, said proudly and persuasively, "Look, mama, muscles!"

Though Andrew was still wetting his pants, he presented his parents with eloquent proof of his successful development. Both Nina and her husband looked at Andrew with adoration and pride.

A YOUNG CHILD IN SEARCH OF GOOD

MARK KERBER was five and one-half years old. He was tall, thin, and lithe as a reed and had short blond hair that stood straight up. All of him was constantly on the move. Mark was passing through the stage in which children are very accommodating. He became very talkative and, seeing my lively interest in his answers, was trying to impress his grandmother, who had accompanied him to the office, and me with his life experiences.

"Grandmother, do you know what?" he addressed her, trying to imitate grown-up talk. "You know what? Our class went to the Brookfield Zoo yesterday. Wow, I saw a cow there! It was so big. I told my teacher we would never be able to afford it!"

"What other animals did you see there?" I dared to interrupt Mark, and delicately tried to get his attention. Mark did not react at first, so I repeated my question. Finally, Mark responded to my question but addressed the answer to his grandmother. He looked at her as he shared this zoological experience. "Grandma, first we saw animals there, but then they took us to see a show and stuff."

"What kind of show did you see there, Mark?" I ventured again.

Interrupted, Mark stopped for an instant, then looked to his grandmother as if asking for sympathy for being tactlessly interrupted, and continued. "Grandma, Grandma, they showed us people in costumes and oceans and trees and brown stuff. These people in costumes, they were working in the ocean. Grandma, the people in the costumes, they were burning the ocean, and they were getting this brown stuff!"

"What brown stuff, what ocean? The ocean does not burn!" I pushed my luck by interjecting another question.

But Mark would not let me into the conversation that easily. He again looked at his grandmother, wanting her to be a witness to the fact that stories are to be told, not to be used as an interview session.

"Grandmother," resumed Mark with increased enthusiasm, "they were burning the ocean and they were getting this brown stuff. The ocean and this brown stuff. They were burning it, and the stuff was all around!"

Mark was totally inspired. His body followed the rhythm of his fervent speech. What was important for him was not what he was telling but his discovery of speech itself, which afforded him the opportunity to establish a bridge between the outside world and the fascinating world inside his mind, inside his unique self.

Through the prism of his vivid imagination he recollected his trip to the Brookfield Zoo, where he must have seen a film about the polluting of the ocean with oil.

Mark visibly savored the chance to be the center of attention for the adults. All excited, he concluded his story with a word of comfort for his grandmother. "Grandmother, don't worry. The people were not real. They were in costumes!" He repeated the last sentence several times to make sure that his grandma heard him.

In his appeal Mark was repeating the universal need that children have to live in a world of values where good is the rule, and evil is only a pretense. Underneath the frightening costume of evil, Mark was trying to find the goodness that he could trust.

WORDS, WORDS, WORDS

I OBSERVED another example of conversation for the sake of conversation when three-year-old Flint arrived at my office for a pre-school exam. Both he and his mother were moderately plump, tall, and energetic people.

Flint talked incessantly and enjoyed every moment of his mono-logue. His emotions were written on his face, and, as if his rich facial expressions did not convey enough, he also tried to express himself with his hands and legs.

It did not take long to realize that what Flint was telling me with an air of great importance was, in reality, all kinds of pleasant, be-nign gibberish. I hoped that our brave, modern judicial system never used him for legal depositions.

On seeing my interest in her child, Flint's mother, Amelda, with a good-humored smile on her face, told me of an episode that had happened the day before. She was walking in a shopping mall, hold-ing onto Flint's hand. Suddenly she felt an outpouring of love for her son.

"Flint, you know what," she said, "I love you."

"Mother, don't be ridiculous!" blurted out her beloved son in re-sponse.

At my request, Amelda asked Flint whether he remembered this episode. He did not. He had simply parroted adult talk, having no idea of the meaning it conveyed.

AN ELOQUENT REQUEST

SIX-YEAR-OLD Nicholas Randy, a smart kid who was a rela-tively new patient of mine, came in with his eight-year-old sister, Wendy, a neatly dressed, pleasant girl with blond hair. Wendy had never been afraid of needles, but Nicholas did not share her attitude. Usually a good-looking child, as are all children at his age, on this day Nicholas was a nervous wreck, with a face twisted in fear and protest. He had come in for his regular school examination, an exam at which immunizations are usually updated, and someone had already warned him of this possible event. His entire appearance said, "I hate shots!"

As his doctor and fellow-citizen I tried to help him out in his time of trouble. "Nicholas," I said, "you have come to a special office. We got rid of shots for your convenience. Nowadays, we don't give shots anymore. We give injections and inoculations."

Having grown wise with experience, Nicholas was not ready "to buy" my innocent attempt at verbal trickery. He continued to express his protest with unrelenting fervor. My eardrums were vibrating with his loud, high-pitched cries.

After I was through examining his courageous sister, I told Nicholas with exalted optimism, "You see, Nicholas, how lucky you are? Your sister gets three shots, and you get *only* one injection!"

Nicholas was far from persuaded. He came back immediately with, "I'd like to get only zero!"

A SEVEN-YEAR-OLD PRODIGY

THE FIRST time I met seven-year-old Dustin Migoni was at the hospital, where he had been admitted by the emergency room with a common diagnosis, "abdominal pain—rule out appendicitis." Our group was on call in the emergency room, and so the case was assigned to us. Since that time, I had seen Dustin on three different occasions in the office and had been continually impressed with his tremendous intelligence, which was combined with hyperactivity and destructive tendencies that, paradoxically, made Dustin more of a slave to, than a beneficiary of, his natural endowment. Dustin had grown up in a broken home; his mother, a woman who had good intentions but who was confused, was herself a manic-depressive and only aggravated Dustin's destructive impulses. This story, however, concerns only my first encounter with Dustin's intelligence when I saw him during my morning rounds in the hospital.

He was a very thin, tall, and somewhat pale child who looked at me with wide-eyed anxiety and with deep distrust. He expected nothing good from me. His mother was not around. Pediatric nurses are usually warm and sensitive people, so I knew Dustin must be really hard to deal with since both the night nurse, who was finishing her shift, and the morning nurse had openly told me about their unhappiness with him.

Dustin had refused all blood tests and injections, and, in the absence of his mother and because it had been impossible to get her on the phone, the medical staff had been reluctant to perform any of the necessary procedures. Now I had arrived and the nurses pinned their hopes of a solution to this problem on me.

It did not take long for me to realize that I was dealing with an intelligent person who had gotten used to controlling others rather than being manipulated by them. Fortunately, Dustin was not seriously ill; he probably had only an intestinal flu, and the tests ordered for him were not an emergency.

After I finished reading the history that the ER physician had taken on Dustin, gave him a physical exam, and wrote up some medical orders, I tried to persuade Dustin to cooperate with us.

"If you want to go home soon, Dustin," I addressed him in my most velvety, persuasive voice, "you had better let us do this stuff right away."

"But *I* would rather wait for my mother," answered Dustin, letting me know by the expression on his animated face that he might start crying at any moment if the circumstances required it.

"Dustin, we need to do these tests for your own benefit. It's in your own best interest," I said, trying to reason with Dustin on his level.

In an instant Dustin started sobbing in the most dramatic manner, and even the walls must surely have felt pity for him.

"I'd really prefer to have my mother to be around me. Will this hurt? How many shots do I need? What is the purpose of all of it?"

Though Dustin's intelligence was amazing, and his words and expressions belonged to a much older child, his behavior and actions were those of a toddler.

Unable to achieve what the nurses expected of me, I again checked his stomach, trying to compensate for the lack of laboratory data with a meticulous physical examination. Dustin's stomach appeared to be very soft, without any signs of tenderness, pain, or discomfort.

"Don't you have any stomach pain? Didn't you complain of stomach pain only four hours ago?" I asked my prodigy patient.

"I never had stomach pain!" Dustin answered with the dignity of a grown-up young man.

"Then why did you complain of it to Dr. Marlin in the emergency room?"

With offended dignity Dustin retorted, "I did not have any pain, for sure. But it hurt me because he was pushing his hand too deep into my stomach."

BEING THIRSTY

ANOTHER CUTE seven-year-old marvel had, with the soundest of logic, easily persuaded his mother he was ill. John Blake's mother, Elizabeth, was very worried because there was a history of diabetes in her family, and she was now afraid that her son had this incurable, chronic disease at his young age.

In the process of taking a history, I learned that all of the members of the family who had diabetes mellitus had contracted it as adults; therefore, the possibility that John had this illness was not great. Children who have diabetes usually suffer from a juvenile form.

As was expected, both blood and urine tests ruled out the possibility of diabetes for now.

Mrs. Blake was pleasantly surprised by the good news but was still unconvinced. "Isn't thirst a sign of diabetes?" she asked me. When I answered affirmatively, she continued in an alarming tone, "In that case, why was it that yesterday, before he went to bed, he told me to wake him up at three o'clock in the morning in order to give him a glass of water? He told me he needed it because otherwise he would get thirsty."

"Mrs. Blake," I objected politely, "if Johnny were really thirsty he would not need to be awakened by you; he would wake up all by himself."

"Yes, Doctor, I follow you," responded Mrs. Blake.

"Ma," interjected little Johnny at this moment. "Why should I wake up by myself? Aunt Millie, she has diabetes too, but Uncle Billy says she sleeps like a log, and snores too."

WITH A LITTLE HELP FROM MY FRIENDS

THE MONTH of August, when the majority of children come in for their school physical, is the pediatrician's busiest time. At this strained time of the year, when each second counts, my thirteen-year-old patient Heidi Mattson came in, accompanied, as she had been for all the preceding visits of the last eleven years, by her mother, Frances. The reason for this visit was Heidi's acne problem.

During the first years of our acquaintance, I had not known how to deal with Frances. She was very demanding and would ask a thousand questions before leaving the office. She also frequently reminded me that her time was valuable and that I should be able to take care of her only daughter without too long a wait. With the passing years I came to realize that Frances did not have anything against me, but, being a punctual person herself, she reasonably expected this of others as well.

It was no surprise when, during a visit the week before, Frances had semijokingly complained that she had waited such a long time she was going to charge me for it.

"It's August, Frances," I answered, trying to apologize for my visitors' long wait. "Believe me, I'm dancing as fast as I can. I haven't even had time to go the washroom." In response, Heidi's mother said only one word—"Go"—but I proudly refused.

Heidi and Frances came in a month later for a follow-up visit. Fortunately, I was not as busy as I had been the previous week. I saw a sly expression on Heidi's face—I have known her so many years that I can read her like a book—and so I understood that she had something in store for me.

"Dr. Tsesis," Heidi said to me respectfully, and I saw mischief in her shining eyes. "Are you sure you don't need to use the washroom?"

In response, I just showed her my fist, which produced joyful laughter from my good friends.

BREAKING THE SHELL

NOT ALL children are endowed with the ability to express themselves. Like clams, such children live within their shell—the shell of the self—and communicate with the external world only poorly at best.

Though Carl Bron was thirteen, his verbal skills were on the level of a well-developed seven-year-old child. He camouflaged this disability by using short, neutral verbal answers that he substituted for more normal speech. I had tried in vain to establish conversations with him.

"Are you are a good student, Carl?"

"Sometimes."

"Do you think your grades will be pretty good this year?"

"You can say so."

"Are your parents OK?"

"Kind of."

"Do you have a girlfriend?"

Suddenly, Carl woke up from his lethargic existence. With unexpected enthusiasm he exclaimed, "Oh, yeah. You bet I do."

UNFORGETTABLE UTTERANCES

DRINKING BEER

SOME PATIENTS stick in memory, even after only one encounter. Twenty-month-old Garrett Piskun, an Alabama boy, was visiting his grandparents, who brought him to my office because of his respiratory allergies. He impressed me with his intelligence in this brief meeting. Seeing Garrett's exhilaration and his urge to communicate, I asked his grandmother to tell me what funny things he had said recently.

While the grandmother was thinking, her alert grandson came to her aid.

"My father drinks beer all night long," he informed me, while his grandmother smiled, visibly embarrassed.

Garrett must have been quite impressed with his father's capacities, because later when I asked him, "Where is your daddy, Garrett?"

he answered with a joyful, "Drinks beer."

To avoid further embarrassment to his grandparents I tried to change the subject.

"What would you like to do, when you grow up?" I asked my visitor.

"I'll bring beer for my daddy," peeped Garrett to me proudly.

STRONG LIKE A BEAK

HOWARD WAS a very cute four-year-old child. To entertain him, I gave him a mask with a duck's beak on it. The yellow beak was made of a firm piece of plastic.

He became very animated when I began imitating the sounds of a duck.

Eventually, he wore the duck's beak on his own nose with enthusiasm. When his mother asked him to take off "the nose," Howard corrected her, telling her that he wore not a nose, but a beak.

"I hope you are going to be healthy and strong," I said to him before leaving the examining room.

"Right," Howard yelled back with a ringing voice. "Strong like a beak!"

DAUGHTER OF A GENIUS

JACQUELINE HUMPHREY brought her four-month-old son in for well-baby visit. Dolly, Jacqueline's six-year-old daughter accompanied the family.

Observing Dolly's shining personality, I could not refrain from remarking on it. "She is a very sweet girl," I said to Jacqueline. Before she could open her mouth to respond Dolly squeaked back, "I know. That's what everybody says."

When I was done with the baby's exam, Jacqueline picked up her beloved son, gave him a kiss, and lovingly said, "You are such a wonderful boy!" Dolly, who was not going to yield her special position in the family, immediately reacted with, "I am also a wonderful boy, right, Ma?" In her determination to be the center of the action, she forgot her gender for a moment.

Looking at both children, I remarked to Jacqueline casually, "They look a lot like your husband."

"Yes. Many people say so," she answered.

I added jocularly, "It looks like your husband's *genes* are stronger than yours."

Immediately little Dolly interjected, "Of course! He is a *genius!*"

BITTEN BY A BANANA

SOMETIMES CHILDREN imagine things which adults might have a hard time following. Five-year-old Kate told me this about her younger brother: "He has a sore throat because a banana bit him."

SOCIAL JUSTICE

TO GIVE children the feeling that they are on their own turf, my office is filled with many toys. Ted Marconi, the son of a local politician, complained to his mother, "It's not fair that my doctor has more toys than I do."

EMBARRASSMENT

TEENAGERS CAN be as good for unforgettable utterances as the younger patients.

Sixteen-year-old Amber Marker came in with complaints typical of an intestinal flu. Amber didn't look very sick despite repeated episodes of vomiting and diarrhea because of this illness. She was of average height and weighed more than 200 pounds.

Though she wore a patient's paper gown, she had not taken off her T-shirt. Overweight children of both sexes are particularly shy about taking off their clothes because they are embarrassed to demonstrate the folds of their bodies, which they would rather hide.

Trying not to offend her modesty, I asked her to remove her T-shirt. "Are you sure?" she asked me, hoping, perhaps, that I might change my mind.

"Yes, I am sure," I answered with an apologetic smile.

She returned the smile to me and then, taking off her gaily colored T-shirt, blurted out with embarrassment, "Pervert."

Her mother, who sat across from us, exclaimed to her daughter, "Amber, this is a doctor!"

Amber replied, "I know Ma, I just can't help it."

NO NEEDLES, NO NEEDLES

THE SCIENCE of psychoanalysis has obtained much rich material by observing the behavior and speech of children. A pediatrician can see it in his own backyard.

Murray, a four-year-old boy, was terrified of getting his vaccinations. "No needles, no needles," he yelled as he hit and scratched his own cheeks with all his might. In front of my eyes I observed an example of the psychic masochism that is described in many books of psychoanalysis.

GUILT

AS BLOOD for an important test was taken from two-year-old Darnell, he cried brokenheartedly, "I am sorry mother, I am sorry mother."

Another child, four-year-old Rosario, had been bitten by the family dog. He rushed to his parents screaming, "It's not me, it's not me. She started it first."

These children, at their young age, already "knew" how to feel guilty.

USING NUMBERS

CHILDREN CONSIDER the ability to use numbers to be a proof of their maturity. Four-year-old Michelle, who likes to discuss family problems with me in a very serious manner, said, "My grandmother is dating Tom because she wants to get married." Then she exclaimed, "Actually, I am a big girl." As she showed me all the fingers on both of her hands, she concluded, "I've got Barbies already. Ten of them."

Children are obsessed with their age, as are many adults. Unlike adults, however, children add years to their age in an attempt to be older. Children like to testify to the number of years old they are by raising their hands and bending their little fingers.

"Guess what, I just turned five because I had my fifth birthday!" bragged little Jonathan.

"I am three—someday I'll be four," Margo revealed to me in a hushed tone that implied a deep secret.

THE ROSES 4

ALL FOUR of the Rose boys were born with a sense of humor and never missed an opportunity to joke, while Mrs. Rose was too busy with her maternal obligations to dwell on the comic side of life. Looking at the Roses 4, as I call them, I sometimes think that they might be the future Marx brothers.

The reason for their visit on this day was the unfortunate fact that eight-year-old Peter was still wetting his bed.

I inquired of Mrs. Rose why she had not told me this problem sooner. "I thought it was Ok," she answered, "because his uncle wet his bed until he was ten."

The Rose brothers immediately picked up on her remark.

"And then he drowned," ten-year-old Freddie finished for her.

"And then he switched to his neighbor's bed." Stan, who was two years older than Freddie, offered his variant.

Everyone laughed.

"And now he does it in his wife's bed," fourteen year old Bud concluded.

Peter laughed along with his brothers. As he was the patient, he had a good excuse for not offering his own version of his uncle's story.

"BYE-BYE 'STITZEZ'"

THE MEMORY of some children's utterances will remain with me forever.

When two-year-old Philip Reed hit his forehead against the corner of a cocktail table while running after a little kitten, he ended up about half an hour later on my examining table getting some stitches. To provide sterility to the operating field, I placed a cover over his face with a small hole to allow the surgery to be performed. As Philip cried piteously and bitterly, he stared at me with a reproachful look through this opening. Tears ran down his cheeks. When everything was over, his mother asked him to thank me, but Philip stubbornly refused.

As I passed by his exam room five minutes later, I could see Philip through the open door. Philip noticed me too and suddenly, in a loud and melodic voice, yelled to me, "Thank you, Doctor!"

A month passed after this visit, and Philip was in the office for a mild cough. He had a scar on his forehead, a reminder of his recent accident. As he looked at me, he touched his scar, which was still sore, and said with gusto, "Bye-bye stitches." "Stitches" in his pronunciation sounded like "stitzez."

For the next couple of months whenever I saw him he told me these "words of courage"—"Bye-bye stitches!"

"DOCTE,DOCTE, DO NOT MAKE ME *HUYT*"

MY MOST cherished memory is of another sweetheart, little Leah. She was three years old when I was removing two plantar warts from her right foot. This procedure, the cutting away of the dead tissue of the warts, was unpleasant for her.

As she repeatedly whimpered, *"Docte, docte,* do not make me *huyt* [hurt]." I saw her head turn in my direction, and the next thing I knew, I felt her soft, wet, baby lips kissing my face.

5

MEMORABLE ENCOUNTERS

Pe-ople of different ages, nationalities, races, and backgrounds; males and females, people who speak different languages; people seeking medical advice and, frequently, a word of support—day in and day out all of these people come to my pediatric office. Each human being, each individual child, is unique and irreplaceable. The life history of each one of them—young and old—would present a huge compendium of memories, emotions, and perceptions that would take many pages to contain. Among these innumerable encounters, some have given me lasting memories.

DOING HIS UTMOST

MANUEL ECHEVERIA, JR., a six-year-old, had been hospitalized for three days; he had been admitted for a fever and hematuria— red blood cells in his urine. He was discharged in good condition with a final diagnosis of hemorrhagic cystitis, meaning that because of a viral infection Manuel's bladder was so inflamed that red blood cells were spilling from its raw internal surface.

Manuel came in for a follow-up visit with his mother and father. Both of his parents, young people around twenty five years old, took good care of their only son. They spoke only Spanish, and Manuel, Jr., at his young age, served as an interpreter for the family.

Manuel Sr., a blue-collar worker, was a stern parent who demanded strict adherence to his rules from his son   rules which

Manuel, Jr., did his best to satisfy. The visit would have been un-eventful except that my patient had difficulty in producing a urine specimen. Because I needed to make sure that the infection was cured and wanted to differentiate it from a more frequent condition, a uri-nary tract infection, it was necessary to perform this urinalysis. After drinking several cups of water, however, and after his mother's per-suasions and his father's scolding, Junior was unable to produce urine, despite his best efforts. When Manuel was finally able to collect some urine, he was in such a hurry to bring it to me for analysis so as to prove to his father that he was a good boy that he managed to trip over his own feet and spill the contents of the plastic cup on the ceramic floor of the washroom.

Manuel's father did not hide his dissatisfaction at his son's awk-ward blunder and ordered him to go back to the washroom and work on a new specimen. Time passed, but Manuel, Jr., did not come out of the bathroom. All of his further efforts to produce urine were un-successful, though he was doing his utmost. I knew this for a fact because, not being aware that he was in one of the washrooms, I had opened the door to an unforgettable scene. Manuel, Jr., with his re-markable black hair sticking out like little hedgehog quills, was stand-ing in front of the toilet bowl with his little spigot in front of an as yet empty urine-specimen container—unable to excrete this biologi-cal fluid.

It was clear that he had spent a long time in this position. Look-ing intently into the cup, he was apparently hoping for the miracle to happen. But the miracle was not happening; the cup remained empty, and a narrow trickle of tears ran from jet black eyes down his olive cheeks.

He saw me standing at the door. Piercing me with eyes filled with guilt, in his lilting Spanish accent Manuel spoke to me in a loud whisper, as if he were sharing his most intimate secret with me, "I'm sorry. I can't pee." Sensing his despair, I told him not to worry: he could provide a specimen the next time he came in. To boost his spirits, I presented him with a set of Crayola markers.

A week later Manuel, Jr., came to my office with his mother. His father was working and was unable to come with them. Manuel, Jr., was scheduled for an early morning appointment, and it was 9:20 a.m. when I entered the room to examine him. As soon as I walked in, without even saying hello to me, Manuel asked in an impatient tone of voice, "Doctor, I would like to know if I could go and pee?" From his disjointed explanation I soon discovered the reason for his urgency. Poor boy. He had not urinated since waking up that morning. He had wanted to be good this time and to provide what he had failed to produce on the previous visit.

He left the room and returned a minute later. With an air of accomplishment, he handed me a container filled to the brim with urine.

His mother smiled proudly, while I, in order to prevent a repetition of the spilled cup episode, carefully took the container from the little hand of my conscientious patient.

MAKE LOVE, NOT WAR

I AM on call every other day; on these days I like to examine my hospitalized patients early in the morning, around 7. At this time, the doctors' lounge is empty, and the hospital corridors are still quiet, as patients are still asleep. Hospital elevators, which later in the day are difficult to catch, are empty and immediately available.

Less human contact results in less stress for me and in some savings of my most valuable commodity—time. A lot of night nurses who become used to the reversed circadian rhythm choose to work nights because this does not burden them with the exhausting routine characteristic of day shifts. At this early hour, patients' charts are not scattered all over the ward unit but are, instead, easy to find. The babies, who are beginning their discovery of the new world, are lying in their cribs and will soon be rolled into their mothers' rooms. In the morning, the traffic on the pediatric floor is minimal, so the nurses might even notice me and give me a detailed report on a newborn's condition. Later, when the nurses are much busier, the report on a newborn might be pared down to a couple of hurried phrases uttered before the nurse rushes off to complete one of her many responsibilities.

On one such early morning, I began my rounds in the newborn nursery of the hospital. The nurse in charge of my patients' care was Monica Judd, a sharp and energetic young woman. Without rushing, she apprised me of the condition of the newborns that were under my care. Eventually, we arrived at a small package wrapped in pinkish blankets that contained a lovely newborn girl with the unusual name (for our newborn nursery) of Rakiya Kagame.

From Monica, I learned that Rakiya was to be breast-fed and that her mother, though she could not speak much English, was doing her best to communicate. The father, however, who was around all the time, would not allow his wife to speak and, instead, continually answered for her. Monica was trying to enlist my support to teach the mother the breast-feeding routine without interference from the father.

Trying to find out if Rakiya's parents spoke any language that I knew, I asked Monica what country they were from. Monica was a good nurse, but geography must not have been a big part of her school curriculum. She frowned, wrinkled her smooth forehead, and, calling over another nurse, Carrie Neil, advised me that the baby's parents were from a country called "Uh, Romania."

"Do you know where Romania is?" she asked Carrie in a businesslike manner.

"Is it somewhere in Asia?" Carrie, who had probably attended the same school as Monica, answered.

I could not allow this geographic speculation to continue and told them that to the best of my knowledge Romania, up to this time, was located in Europe. After Monica and Carrie politely agreed with my qualified statement, I gave an attentive look to my very young patient and came to the conclusion that it was pretty unlikely that her parents were from Romania.

"Her parents cannot be from Romania," I pronounced. "There are a lot of people in Eastern Europe, but I have never heard of any people with dark skin living there. Try something else."

Monica began her deep thinking process again. "I know it sounds something like Row. . .," she said finally with a disarming smile.

"Oh, Rhodesia. But it is called Zimbabwe now. It's in Africa!" I exclaimed "I've never met anybody from there. Very interesting."

As expected, my examination of baby Rakiya confirmed my impression of her excellent health. I wrote a note in her medical record and went to Room 513 to bring the good news to Rakiya's parents.

As I entered the room, Maquiba Kagame, who only five hours earlier had delivered the baby, was involved in a lively conversation with her husband, Faustin, who stood next to her bed.

Both parents were in their early thirties. Maquiba was somewhat plump, which made her pleasant face even more attractive. Faustin was slim and very agile.

At any place on the globe, good mothers of all colors and nationalities have features in common. These universal characteristics have been celebrated by poets and composers since time immemorial. For Maquiba, to be a mother was as natural as to breathe air in order to live. A maternal glow radiated from her face. She lived in a world of unconditional love and care for her new child. As I walked in, the couple stopped talking and looked expectantly at me. I introduced myself and told both parents the good news about their daughter's condition.

It soon became clear to me why Faustin did most of the talking. He was not trying to dominate the conversation as Monica had thought, but Maquiba's poor English forced him to take an active role in the dialogue.

As I started to talk with Mr. and Mrs. Kagame, I learned that, five months earlier, Maquiba had come to the United States with their three older children. Her husband had arrived two months before that.

On hearing that Mr. Kagame had his own business, which represented the interests of several companies from his country, I remarked that I was not aware that Zimbabwe had a significant amount of industry. Faustin's face made it clear that he knew nothing of Zimbabwe.

I was unable to identify the accent that prevented me from understanding him. On the other hand, he was having difficulty understanding my Russian accent. As a result I couldn't figure out what country the family was from. Unable to grasp the name of the country Mr. Kagame was giving, I asked him what the capital city of his country was.

"Oh, Rwanda," I exclaimed, after Faustin replied that the capital of his country was Kigali.

Our conversation, which took place before the French military forces arrived to establish some order in that country, concerned the civil war and the ensuing anarchy and famine that plagued Rwanda at that time. Faustin, after graduating from college in England in 1989, had worked in Kigali as an electrical engineer. Facing the catastrophic chain of events occurring in his country, he decided to move to the United States to live with his brother Najib in Chicago. He arrived in Chicago intending to send for his wife and children as soon as possible.

I asked him about the war in his country, and he explained to me that the war in Rwanda was not among political and economical groups, but among different tribes.

"It will never stop," Faustin expressed his opinion in a prophetic tone, "until the last tribes kill one another. The famine is everywhere. The majority of the people are hungry, and many of them are dying from starvation. On the other hand, there is enough ammunition to continue the fighting for the next twenty years."

"Where did they get all these weapons?" I asked.

"Oh, our country received them on a generous scale from all over the world. Everybody was happy to sell them to us, to assure that we could kill each other."

"How did you get your family here to the United States?"

"I left my wife with our children in Kigali until she called me and told me that there was no hope left for our country. Her older sister had been killed for a piece of bread two weeks earlier. My brother and I collected all of our money and went to Kigali. A week later we returned to Chicago, and the family was united."

"Did your wife belong to the same tribe as you?" I asked. "No," he said and then translated the question to his wife who had been attentively listening to our conversation. Then, as if he had read my thoughts, Faustin, looking with love at his wife's innocent face, said, "In Rwanda we would fight each other, and I might kill her there." He translated this statement to Maquiba and, with a mischievous smile, pretended to bend a bow with an imaginary arrow aimed at his wife. Maquiba did not need to have this gesture explained. She understood it instantly and smiled widely in response.

"Do you know the expression 'Make love, not war?'" I inquired of Faustin. He looked at me, trying to get the meaning of the words, and repeated them twice. In a moment he understood their meaning and immediately translated to Maquiba. They both laughed infectiously.

"Doctor, you are right, Faustin said. "This expression is precisely about us. I like it a lot!"

THE UGLY DUCKLING

ONE DAY in August office established the record for the most patients we had ever examined in a day. August, as I've mentioned, is a special month for pediatricians, as this is the month that most of the physical exams for schools and daycare centers are performed. I came home late that August evening and was completely exhausted; the last thing I wanted was a call from the emergency room where I was on duty that night.

The worst medical emergencies always seem to happen in the middle of the night. Sure enough, the phone rang at two o'clock on this morning. As I picked up the receiver, I hoped it was one of those easy-to-handle-over-the-phone-type of calls or, better still, a wrong number. Alas, it was neither; it was a real emergency. In these situations, the words of a former pediatrician who was a longtime friend of mine come to mind. Whenever I asked if she had seen any unusual medical cases recently, she invariably answered, "Vladimir, I hate interesting cases!"

Harvey DeBari, an emergency room physician, called to inform me that he was admitting a twelve-year-old patient named Shonice Kanley, who was presenting dangerous signs of a diabetic pre-coma. The patient's name did not tell me anything; her family had just signed up for my services through a health maintenance organization, and Shonice had never visited my office.

According to Harvey, Shonice was in serious trouble: her blood glucose level was more than 500 (almost five times higher than normal), and she had large amounts of sugar in her urine and a large quantity of acetone in her blood and urine—signs of a serious metabolic derangement that can precede and accompany a diabetic coma. In these circumstances each minute is precious. I told Harvey that I was on my way to the emergency room and asked no more questions.

My wife had instantly understood the situation and hastily prepared my clothes for me before I hung up the phone; they lay in a heap in front of me waiting to be put on. In an instant the exhaustion that I had felt a moment before was transformed into a flowing stream of bubbling energy.

Fifteen minutes later, with the adrenaline rushing through my body after having run red lights and stop signs, I reached the emergency room, where I found Shonice Kanley. She had wires and tubes attached to her body and looked very frightened. Her mother, Shirley Kanley, sat next to her.

Though Shonice was only twelve years old, she weighed more than 200 pounds. Exhaustion and fear were written on her round face. Luckily, she was not in a real coma but in a pre-coma; that is, she was fully conscious, but her respiration pattern hinted at a Kussmaul type of breathing, a certain sign of coma. Her basic vital signs, heart rate, blood pressure, and temperature, were all in the normal range.

Shonice's mother was very friendly and cooperative, though it was clear that she was extremely concerned for her daughter's health. I learned from her that though Shonice had been overweight since a very young age, she had never been sick before. A month and a half earlier Shonice had begun to complain of a lack of energy and, though she had been a good student, she stopped performing well at school.

Shonice lay with her eyes closed, opening them from time to time to look at both of us as we talked. She was unable to participate in the conversation even if she had wanted to—she was much too sick.

Soon after I finished Shonice's history and physical, my favorite diabetes specialist, Sam Zussman, whom I had called for a consultation, came in to examine Shonice. Sam is a fine example of professional expertise and good bedside manners. He is always immediately available for critical clinical cases. It was a comfort to see his tall, slightly stooped figure with his Littman stethoscope hanging from his long neck. He knew how important his presence was at this moment and, although it was three o'clock in the morning, I could see an expression of professional satisfaction on his face.

Sam greeted me, and I told him all I knew about our patient; we then went through the results of the lab tests and began to discuss a treatment plan. Our common feeling was that Shonice's condition was stable enough to allow her to be admitted to the regular pediatric floor rather than the intensive care unit, as had been initially thought.

Finally, I could speak to my patient. Knowing how stressful the situation must be for her, I wanted to calm her down and to encourage her. I told her that she would soon be feeling much better and that the process of improving her condition had already started with the treatment she was receiving. Shonice's large, bubblelike body occupied the entire width of the ER cart, and she looked completely lost—she definitely needed as much emotional help as she could get. She was listening to me, but her condition prevented her from talking.

"Is Shonice usually shy and quiet?" I asked Mrs. Kanley. She gave an affirmative reply and added that besides being shy and quiet, her daughter was also humble and modest as well.

I spent another ten minutes in conversation with Shonice, telling her that she should not worry, that the doctors and nurses would provide her with the best possible care. "And one of these days, Shonice, you may become a doctor or a nurse. Guess what? You yourself would then be one of the people who treat and help children with problems similar to yours!"

To my surprise, I noticed a brief, incredulous, though scarcely perceptible smile on Shonice's face. She looked at me and said weakly but thoughtfully, "Thank you." A moment later she dozed off.

Shonice's condition improved. Four days after her admission she was discharged home, supplied with a pile of books and instructive materials to teach her how to take care of her diabetes.

After Shonice was discharged from the hospital, Dr. Zussman and I took care of her health problems on an outpatient basis. I regularly received professional letters from Sam that updated me on Shonice's health.

The Kanley family had come from Haiti a couple of years before this when Mrs. Kanley's former husband had demanded divorce after fifteen years of marital life. After the divorce Mrs. Kanley decided to begin a new life and, taking all four of her children, went to her sister, who lived in the United States.

The family settled in a suburb of Chicago in which the majority of the people belonged to the blue-collar middle class. The village had a very good school system.

Shonice was the eldest child and had two brothers and a sister. Anytime her mother brought in any of the children, together or separately, she always updated me on Shonice's condition.

Initially, Shonice came to my office for regular visits every three to six months. Her mother always accompanied her, and, though I tried to talk directly to my patient, Mrs. Kanley did most of the talking, while Shonice remained reserved and modest. On several occasions I invited Shonice to talk more actively and even suspected that she had some problem with her verbal skills, but her mother told me repeatedly with her reassuring smile that Shonice was a good student.

There are two types of diabetes—juvenile and mature. Though the juvenile type usually begins in childhood, and the mature type begins at an older age, both of these forms can occur in any age group. Unfortunately, the juvenile type of diabetes carries a significantly worse prognosis in terms of the course of the disease and its complications. One year after Shonice's hospitalization I received a letter from Dr. Zussman that informed me that, luckily for Shonice, though her symptoms had started at the age of twelve years, she suffered not from the juvenile but from the mature type of diabetes.

Shonice and her mother came in soon after I had received this letter, and although both of them seemed happy about the news from Dr. Zussman, Mrs. Kanley displayed this happiness more openly than her daughter. Only at the end of the visit did I see a happy smile on Shonice's face, and her handshake, which was usually very careful and bashful, was firm and unhesitating.

Another year passed. I was happy to observe that Shonice's body had started to grow in height, and though she was not losing weight, she was not gaining it, either. Eventually, her appearance began to take on a more normal shape instead of her former bubblelike contour. To my amazement, Shonice was becoming not only attractive but elegant as well.

Six months later we congratulated each other on a new, exciting event in Shonice's life. With the new proportions of her body, her body fat relative to her height had been reduced, and she no longer needed insulin to control her diabetes. This confirmed once more that Shonice had the mature, not the juvenile type of diabetes; this type could be controlled by diet and, instead of injections of insulin, by a medication taken orally in tablet form once a day.

Since Shonice stopped needing injections of insulin, she came to my office only once a year for an exam. Four years passed, and on another summer day she came to my office without her mother. She had driven herself—after all Shonice was now eighteen years old. At this age even the most dedicated parents usually stop accompanying their offspring to the doctor's office. She had grown taller since I last saw her, and though she was still plump, she was far from being morbidly obese as she had been the first time I met her.

Whereas it had once been a depressing sight to see Shonice—a human being who had lost all of the contours of a healthy human body—I now saw a proportionally built, healthy young woman.

"Okay, Shonice, what brought you in today?" I asked.

In the past Shonice had always been shy and embarrassed with me; today, surprisingly, Shonice's soft voice sounded strong and proud. With no trace of embarrassment, she told me that she had come to the office to have a physical examination for college.

"College?" I asked in surprise but then immediately realized that my patient was indeed of college age. Eighteen years! Six years had passed like an instant. "What college are you going to attend, Shonice?"

Shonice looked straight at me and answered briskly in one breath, "Yale."

"Yale! I knew you were a good student but never realized you were so good! That's great! What are you going to study there, Shonice?"

Shonice did not answer right away. I saw a solemn expression on her face. She had something important to tell me. "I want to become a specialist who treats children with diabetes," she finally said, as if this were a statement she had been preparing in her mind for a long time.

"Do you remember, Shonice, what I told you once, the first time we met?" I asked her. "Didn't I tell you that you would be Ok and that you would never need to go to the hospital as long as you took good care of your condition? You've made it!"

"Right," she answered, and in a lowered tone of voice she said, "You also told me then that one of these days I would be helping children who have the same problem I have."

"Boy, you remember this!" I exclaimed, not expecting that she would remember words addressed to her at a time when she was so critically ill.

"Besides, I don't need to take insulin anymore. I just watch my diet. I've also been losing weight all this time," continued Shonice, this time with a challenging tone in her voice, while I was signing her papers.

At this moment I realized that she expected me to be more attentive to her accomplishments, which for her meant more than just her acceptance to Yale University

She achieved her desired effect: I felt guilty for not being sensitive enough to my longtime patient. Looking at Shonice as she was ready to leave, I told her, "I bet you've lost at least fifty pounds!"

She looked at me with triumph. Suddenly, a big childish smile spread across her face, exposing dazzling white teeth.

"Sixty-five!" she exclaimed, as if she were taunting me, "and my father made up with my mother. He came from Haiti and lives with us. We are one family again."

She received a completed and signed medical form from me and left the examining room to head toward life's horizon.

THE POWER OF HYPNOSIS

WHILE WORKING as a pediatrician in Odessa, Ukraine, in the early 1970s, I, like many of my colleagues, was forced to supplement my meager salary. I worked part-time as a sports-medicine physician at a sports club called Locomotive. At that time the club boasted the Soviet Olympic kayak team among its membership, including the late Olga Ryabchynskaya, who became an Olympic champion at the Munich competition.

My boss, Dr. Brotman, was demonstrating his enthusiasm for the application of various psychological methods, including hypnosis, as an aid to athletic achievement. I did not think very highly of his abilities as a hypnotist—the athletes were opening their eyes and talking and chuckling when Dr. Brotman wasn't looking in their direction. Thus, each party was just pretending to be doing the right thing. I challenged my boss on this, and with help of my colleagues and several books on medical hypnosis I learned in about three months how to hypnotize subjects to produce a positive therapeutic effect.

The pediatric office is not well suited for using hypnosis as a method of treatment because a hypnotic session takes so much longer than prescribing procedures and medications; thus, I do not use medical hypnosis very frequently. The technology of medicine has gradually overtaken the art of medicine: unsophisticated parents and patients have more faith in the material symbols of treatment—machines, injections, tablets—than in the power of the human word and human intuition.

Hypnosis, however, belongs to a type of medicine that can, in some cases produce truly miraculous results. One such case is enuresis, nighttime bed-wetting, a condition that can persist into the late teen years. Sometimes, when it is obvious to me that hypnosis could be effective in the treatment of enuresis, especially when it might be more effective than conventional methods of treatment, I feel obliged to offer it.

Mrs. Lipkins had two children, Teron and Yvonne. Despite his large frame, which accommodated more than 170 pounds, and his reputation for being an outstanding athlete, Teron, at twelve years of age, was still unable to reliably control his bladder. At least every other night he would awaken to find himself in a wet bed.

The drug therapies that are available for the treatment of enuresis are meant to be used only temporarily, not forever. Sooner or later, with the development and maturation of the patient's neuroregulatory mechanisms, he or she attains control of the urinary bladder sphincter. With or without treatment the majority of children are able to attain control over their bladder by the age of twelve. One of the important purposes of drug therapy is to boost the morale of the patient and patient's parents by demonstrating that the bed-wetting problem is transitory.

For those few children who still have this problem after age twelve, one way of helping them to bypass their slow progress is to appeal to their ego, their self, through hypnosis. This appeal might produce a strong effect and give a powerful impetus of motivation to help them gain control over their bodily functions. When the rapport between the hypnotist and the person under hypnosis is strong, the hypnotic suggestion is even more powerful. At twelve years of age, Teron was mature enough to handle this challenge to his self. When I offered to try hypnosis on Teron, Mrs. Lipkins and her son both agreed without hesitation. Teron had nothing to lose. He was very shy and reserved for a child of his age for he had been living with strong feelings of shame and guilt because of his inability to gain control over this important physiological act.

Thus, I did most of the talking while Teron answered me in short, simple sentences and bit his lower lip in embarrassment. A small smile appeared on his face when I told him about the possibility of good results.

Teron had been born in Missouri; he had a heavy southern accent that made some of his phrases and words difficult for me to understand. I'm sure he had the same problems with my Slavic-Midwestern American accent, and so I tried to speak slowly and clearly to ensure that Teron understood the psychological terms I was using.

Fortunately, Teron was quite a hypnotizable subject; he must have inherited this quality from his mother—on several occasions during the session, I had to shake her and wake her up so she didn't fall off her chair. After a short introduction my patient was in a deep hypnotic sleep. On awakening, Teron told me that he did not remember what I had said during the session but that he felt good. After three more sessions Teron demonstrated a steady and definite improvement.

Teron and his mother came to the office for the fourth hypnotic session, and I saw a contented expression on both of their faces. They thanked me for the good results that Teron had with the treatment: Teron had his first sleepover at a friend's house. In the morning he woke up in a splendidly dry bed.

After such an achievement Teron was undergoing a noticeable transformation—his expression of guilt and embarrassment disappeared, he stopped avoiding eye contact with me, and he participated more actively in conversations. He was behaving like a normal twelve-year-old. Teron approached me and, in his lovely southern accent, thanked me. We firmly shook hands and got to work.

When hypnosis works, on each subsequent session the subject tends to go into a deeper stage of sleep. This is exactly what happened to Teron during the fourth session. By the same token, his mother was more prone to the hypnotic suggestion as well—my time was divided between waking her up and continuing to maintain her son in his deep sleep.

The high degree of hypnotic sleep that Teron had attained allowed me to use a new method of intervention in this session, that might otherwise have awakened him in the process of its application. This method consisted of making Teron himself restate the hypnotic suggestion that I was presenting to him. Trying to be clear and accurate, I told Teron what was expected of him and then asked him to repeat back my suggestion word-for-word.

At my request Teron slowly brought back the normal muscle tone of his relaxed mouth. In a unique combination of southern Missouri and Russian accents he obediently vocalized, "I am going to be dry in bed. I vill never be vet again. I vill be vonderfull. I vill be vell."

Fully awakened by this speech, Mrs. Lipkins listened to her son with complete incredulity. Though she could understand my Russian accent, the same accent coming from her son's mouth was bewildering to her. She gave me a dubious look.

Fortunately, when Teron woke up, his mother could again hear his colorful southern accent. His Russian enunciation was locked away in one of the drawers of his subconscious.

Before Mrs. Lipkins left the exam room I asked her whether she had been worried that her son would start talking like a foreigner.

"I don't care what accent Teron talks with," Mrs. Lipkins answered with a sunny smile on her face, "as long as he doesn't pee in his bed."

PUZZLES OF MIND

A PEDIATRICIAN frequently has more problems communicating and dealing with the parents of his patients than with the patients themselves. A special challenge is presented when the parent's mind does not function in the familiar system of reasoning in which effect follows cause.

Cynthia Jefferson, a middle-aged woman with an expressive, determined, sharply angled face brought in her eleven-year-old daughter, Laura, in with an unusual request. To make sure I understood her correctly, I asked her to repeat this request three times. Ms. Jefferson wanted to have her daughter evaluated "with blood tests," because she suspected that someone was trying to poison Laura's food. Laura, who was quite an active and unruly child, did not appear to be at all sick. On the contrary, while her mother spoke to me, Laura was running around in circles to burn off some of her extra energy. Laura's hectic behavior did not arouse any reaction from her mother.

I asked Cynthia what made her think that her daughter was being poisoned. She sighed and in a low but determined voice told me that, besides her daughter, she herself was a victim of premeditated poisoning. According to Ms. Jefferson, whenever she and Laura visited a restaurant, they were given food that was poisoned. She began noticing this alarming pattern about a month earlier. She had written a letter about her suspicions and findings to the president of the manufacturing company where she worked as a secretary.

I knew that it was impossible to dissuade Cynthia from her suspicions—she required professional mental help, however, I wanted to have a better idea to what degree Cynthia's mind was distorted. I asked her why waitresses from restaurants that were located in different suburbs would be interested in harming her and how they would coordinate their actions. She looked at me with pity. "It is not difficult to understand at all," she told me with reproach in her voice. "All that's necessary is a telephone call. It's a plot."

Cynthia's mind was preoccupied with the plot to poison her and her daughter. At Cynthia's office they knew how serious she was about these suspicions; she showed me the letter she had written to her boss. This letter was grammatically impeccable but lacked any logic. I wondered what impression Cynthia's superiors at the manufacturing company had formed when they read this wild letter.

On the other hand, I felt a responsibility for doing something in the face of Cynthia's paranoia. What if something happened to her or her child while she was driving her car? Alas, I could not do too much for her—until a person who has a mental disease puts himself or herself in real jeopardy or asks for help, it is impossible to force such a person to obtain a consultation with a mental health specialist.

Cynthia planned to drive from my office for an appointment with Dr. Einberg, her primary physician. Thinking that he might be more successful than I could be in helping Cynthia, I phoned him, but, instead of interest, this produced only irritation and displeasure on his part—he was too busy for this request.

Maybe the police could do something, I thought. I told Cynthia that with such a serious case she should take the food that might be poisoned to the police or the FBI. I thought that her request would arouse suspicion on their part and that they had a better chance of forcing Cynthia to undergo a psychiatric evaluation.

"Doctor, are you crazy?" Cynthia said, "Don't you understand that they are in league with the waitresses all over?" I apologized for my naiveté.

Ms. Jefferson was a single mother, and her parents lived in another state, so I did not have a real chance to talk to anyone about her problem. After Cynthia left my office, I tried to call her at her home on several occasions, but no one ever answered her phone.

A couple of months later Ms. Jefferson appeared in my office again. I was glad to hear that this time her concern about Laura's health was nothing exotic. Laura was coughing and had a sore throat and a mild fever—the usual staple of the pediatric diet.

As on the first visit, Cynthia did not create an unfavorable impression. She was neatly dressed, friendly, and lively. Everything she told me this time, however, was logical and reasonable.

At a suitable moment, I gently asked her what had happened with the conspiracy to poison her and her daughter that had preoccupied her so much on the previous visit.

"Oh, that," she said in a convinced voice, looking at a door at the same time. "No problem at all. We simply do not go out to eat. I have been fixing food at home since then."

I expressed my satisfaction with this constructive solution to the problem and in conclusion handed Ms. Jefferson a prescription for her daughter's cough.

Ms. Jefferson listened attentively to my instructions. When I finished my explanations, she asked, with a determined expression on her face, "Doctor, can she take only one medicine, not two?"

"Why only one, not two?"

"Well, Doctor," replied Ms. Jefferson, who then smiled at me as if to someone who should know more than most about her considered judgment, "because I do not want my daughter to become a hypochondriac."

A VOODOO STORY

THE MINUTE I came into the exam room, where Betty Crandall, a middle-aged single mother, was waiting for me, I felt there was an invisible, high-voltage energy emitting from her apprehensive face.

Betty had accompanied her eight-year-old daughter, Hannah, to my office, and her mother's nervous tension was reflected on her face, as well. Though Hannah looked like a normal child, an experienced observer would sense in her an anxiety of an existential kind—the result of the child's exposure to psychological factors that were interfering with the joie de vivre of her childhood. There was a pronounced irritation around her lips, in medical lingo a "perilabial inflammation," which was caused by her continual licking of her lips—the physical testimony to her internal tension. As with any other ticlike condition that accompanies a significant degree of emotional stress, people who have a lip-licking problem are not aware that they have it.

Many ticlike conditions disappear by themselves and can be ignored. In Hannah's case, however, the constant touching of her lips with her tongue had produced such an acute soreness that it could not be disregarded. The condition had to be brought to the child's attention so that her conscious mind could try to control this unconscious action.

I took a mirror in my left hand, put my right arm around Hannah's shoulders, and turned her head toward the mirror. At this moment I felt Hannah lean her small body toward me in a trusting and natural way, as if we were father and daughter. Like innumerable children in her predicament, Hannah's human heart was yearning to have both a mother and a father.

The stress of life had also left its imprint on her mother's face. Betty was working as a dietician in a nursing home. She looked thin and emaciated; her appearance reminded me of a victim of starvation or of AIDS in its active stage or of someone who is a heavy abuser of alcohol or drugs. The reason for her appearance, however, was not physical—she was suffering from emotional problems. A long history of betrayed hopes and expectations was written on Ms. Crandall's face, though she still retained the attractive look of her youthful age.

I had met Ms. Crandall and her daughter on several occasions, but I had never had a chance to speak with Betty for very long. I knew, however, that she liked to talk.

"It looks like you are going through a lot of tension, Ms. Crandall. The majority of people with weight problems need to lose weight, but you need to gain it immediately. Are you worried a lot?"

"Yes," she answered, showing gratitude for my interest in her condition. "It's all here," she added, pointing to her chest and stomach, "I just don't feel I want to eat. Worries, too many worries, Doc!"

Seeing my sincere interest, she continued to tell me that she was distressed by the fact that her ex-husband had recently met her boyfriend, a professional football player whom she was now dating, and might tell him compromising facts about her. This, from her standpoint, was the reason her boyfriend had refused to see her recently.

"Now, Hannah and I are afraid that my boyfriend, the football player, might never return to me."

After a short comment on Betty's amorous perturbations, I noted to her that she did not help her daughter's tensions by involving her in her private problems—Hannah had enough pressures of her own.

Betty gave me a look of astonishment. Apparently it had never occurred to her that she could affect her daughter negatively by taking her on as a companion on her exhausting roller-coaster ride of worries and apprehensions. Encouraged by her positive reaction, I screwed up my courage and asked her whether, with all the physical and emotional distress she was going through, she was seeking some help from a psychiatrist or psychologist.

Betty answered that she was undergoing some counseling with a psychologist, but she was becoming disappointed with her lack of success. She was now looking into religion as a way to ease her emotional problems. This had begun two months ago when her former boyfriend, the one before the football player, told her that a drink he had given her had a voodoo curse on it.

Since then, though "by birth" she was a Methodist she had become involved with, and fascinated by, voodoo rituals. She and her eight-year-old daughter had been attending voodoo assemblies on a regular basis for the past two months.

There was nothing I could really do about Betty's romance with voodoo. With sadness and pain, I looked at her daughter, who was destined because of her mother's "help" to share in the many confusions of the modern world. If Ms. Crandall were physically abusing her daughter, I could call a protective agency and immediately receive appropriate support. But when a child's mind is being poisoned and disturbed by superstition and a lack of rationality—which can be much more dangerous than physical abuse—I can do nothing. Betty's right to choose the course of Hannah's upbringing was protected by the tenets of a democratic state.

I felt, as I have at other times in similar situations, like a passenger in a train, observing another train slowly but relentlessly moving in the opposite direction. I could see what was happening in there, exchange a few words, even make suggestions to the passengers of the other train, but could change almost nothing.

Not everything is in our hands.

MRS. CORRY SAVES THE FAMILY JEWELS

MARTIN CORRY and his mother came to my office together for a follow-up visit after surgery Martin had at a local hospital. Mrs. Corry told me this story.

Martin, who was eleven years old, had developed a sudden pain in his left testicle during gym class. His mother was immediately notified, and she arrived at the school within fifteen minutes, at which time the paramedics were putting Martin on a stretcher and taking him to the hospital.

In another fifteen minutes Mrs. Corry was sitting next to her son who had been placed on a gurney in one of the numerous exam rooms of a suburban hospital's emergency room. Martin, who was not usually a complainer, was now whining and crying with severe pain.

A nurse who was busily chewing on a piece of gum in a business-like manner, not forgetting to crack it at regular intervals, hardly looked at Martin as she took his temperature and filled out medical forms.

Then an ER physician, a young man with rosy cheeks and a diamond earring in his left ear, thoroughly examined Martin.

"Most probably a twisted testicle, testicle torsion, a surgical condition." He shortly summarized these observations.

He left Martin and came back in five minutes. "I spoke with Dr. Boikin, a urologist," he informed Mrs. Corry. "He trusts my diagnosis, but before he operates on your son he wants to have a blood test and a Doppler scan done."

"How long will this take?" asked Mrs. Corry. She felt that her heart was being pierced by her son's crying and moaning.

She was told that it was out of the hands of those in ER to predict the exact time—it was up to the lab and the Medical Image Department—but that they in the ER would do their best. The procedures had already been requested. Besides, Dr. Boikin was operating on another patient at the moment, so no time was being lost by waiting.

The laboratory technician took Martin's blood, but thirty minutes passed and no one had showed up from the Medical Image Department.

Martin's pain was getting worse. He was periodically screaming from it, while wiping the tears that ran down his face with the sleeve of his shirt.

Both the ER physician and the nurse who were caring for Martin were faithfully following Dr. Boikin's medical orders. Every day they hear children crying, and there was nothing new about a mother pleading for more extensive care for her child. Besides, they were busy with other patients—somebody came in with a severe bronchial asthma attack, someone else was brought in after a car accident, somebody was bleeding. Sooner or later all the patients are taken care of.

Forty-five minutes had passed since Martin was admitted to the ER. Mrs. Corry, though soft-spoken, was a woman of action; she again tried to bring attention to her son's condition.

"My son is in severe pain—can you do something for him?" she asked the nurse.

The emergency room of the suburban hospital was large and spacious. Martin was placed in partition number six at the far end of the unit. The sounds of the crying that was breaking his mother's heart dissolved in the spacious air of the ER, which was filled with all of the sounds produced by other sick people.

"Please wait, Mrs. Corry. They are on their way," answered the nurse quickly, not looking at Mrs. Corry; then, cracking her gum, she ran to another patient.

Mrs. Corry suddenly realized the futility of her efforts to speed up the course of medical intervention for her son. For the nurse, Martin was "the patient from bed six," but for his mother, he was her son. She was in an ER with a full medical staff, but she felt as if she were in a desert. The fluorescent lights reflected off the impeccably clean tile floor, and numerous machines were buzzing; what was absent were the human elements, like compassion and sensitivity, which are not a part of medical technology and for which no insurance carrier provides payment.

Another fifteen minutes passed, but still nothing happened. Martin was shaking with his unrelenting pain. At that moment Mrs. Corry saw a man wearing the uniform of a private ambulance company; he was leaving the ER after having brought in a patient.

"Mister," she called to him, hoping that he would answer.

To her surprise he answered her in a normal, friendly way.

"Sir, how much would it cost to get you to drive my son to Doctors' Community Hospital?" she inquired.

"A hundred and fifty bucks."

"Ok. Can you wait for me outside, please?" asked Mrs. Corry, as she hurriedly handed the man a check.

"No problem, ma'am. See you later."

Mrs. Corry returned to her son and in a soft but determined tone told him that they should leave. Martin slowly picked up his hurting body, and, limping and holding onto his sore crotch, he followed her.

The ER personnel were too busy with other patients. Martin, though seriously sick, did not, as far as they were concerned, require immediate care.

Nobody paid attention to the patient "from bed six," who was walking out of the ER, supported by his mother. Nobody noticed them. Unobstructed, they left.

Fifty feet from the entrance to the ER a private medical ambulance was waiting for them with its motor running. The door was flung open, two strong men placed Martin on a stretcher, the sirens sounded, and the ambulance raced toward Doctors' Community Hospital. About ten minutes later the ambulance had reached its destination; half an hour later Martin was in the operating room. The surgery was successful.

In the surgical waiting room the urologist who had performed the surgery on Martin told Mrs. Corry that the boy had gotten the operation just in time.

That is how Mrs. Corry saved her son's testicle.

Did Mrs. Corry do the right thing? That is a hard question. She acted on impulse, guided by her maternal instinct. Her main motivating force was her inability to passively observe the suffering of her child. Fortunately for Martin and for her, Doctors' ER was not busy that night, and the people who happened to be working that particular shift took Martin's suffering close to their hearts, as it should be.

It all depends on people. Nonprofessional and professional alike.

SOME LIKE IT TWISTED

MRS. MELODY MCDONALD, a thin woman with a pleasant appearance who was in her early thirties, was an executive in one of the largest Chicago insurance companies. She came to our office for the first time to bring in her son for his well-baby visit. Her two-week-old son, Andrew, was cute, cuddly, and healthy.

The physical examination of my little patient proceeded in the regular order: step by step, from top to bottom. Andrew appeared to be perfectly normal until I came to the examination of his genitals. At that time I saw an abnormality that I had never encountered before: Andrew's uncircumcised penis, which was normally developed, instead of being oriented in the regular position where the urethral opening on the head of the penis is pointing straight forward, was rotated, as was the rest of the penis, exactly ninety degrees counter-clockwise around its longitudinal axis. Despite my assiduous attempts to bring it to a regular position, it stubbornly kept turning toward the internal surface of the left thigh.

Trying to be as delicate and tactful as possible, I let Melody know about my finding, reassuring her that the problem did not appear to be serious. "Your next well-baby visit is in two weeks; let's reexamine Andrew then," I said. "Hopefully, it is just a transitory problem."

Two weeks later, Mrs. McDonald was back in the office with her firstborn son. Alas, the penis continued to face in the wrong direction, resolutely refusing to be placed in the proper position.

"It looks, Mrs. McDonald, like we need to consult with a pediatric urologist about your son. I am sure that the position of your son's penis will by no means, now or in the future, impede his urinary or sexual functions. The problem is rather cosmetic and, if I may say so, of careful aim during the emptying of the bladder. It is unusual, indeed, to have a penis turned almost ninety degrees from its normal position."

To my surprise, Mrs. McDonald was listening to my words not only without any visible enthusiasm but with some degree of, if not resentment, then estrangement. She was gazing fixedly at her son, disengaging from her steady eye contact with me.

Unable to understand her disinterest, I continued. "Let me personally call a pediatric urologist of your or my choosing for an appointment. He will help us decide what would be the best course of action for Andrew's problem."

I still did not see a positive reaction from Melody, who appeared to be a cooperative mother. Maybe she did not really understand what I was talking about. I started to worry.

Taking a piece of paper, I made rough sketches in two projections of the position of a normal penis and the position of her son's penis.

When I finished my artistic exercise, I felt that I must have inadvertently perpetrated a tactless blunder. Though Mrs. McDonald was nodding her head to show that she followed my explanation, she was blushing and hiding her eyes from me and avoided looking at the sketch as if I had drawn "a dirty" picture. Whether it was because of her natural bashfulness or because of her modest upbringing, I did not know, but as quickly as I could, I removed the sketch from the desk, threw it in the wastepaper basket, and finished the visit with a blithe remark that the pediatric urologist who would soon examine Andrew would help all of us to put our mind at ease about the deviation of Andrew's private part.

The next well-baby appointment for Andrew was scheduled in a month. He arrived for this appointment accompanied by his happily married parents. Mr. Stanley McDonald, whom I had never met before, impressed me with his good-natured appearance and his well-built body, which rippled with imposing muscles. Though he was an accountant, his build and towering height made him look like a player for the NBA.

Andrew, as on the previous visits, was in excellent health. Knowing that by this time he should already have been examined by the specialist, I started to look for a consultation report, meticulously turning over each sheet in his medical record. The report was not in the baby's file.

"Mrs. McDonald, was your son examined by the urologist?" I finally asked Melody. She did not reply, and then, not saying a word, she shook her head to indicate that Andrew had not yet been examined by a specialist.

Both McDonalds produced a favorable impression—they were nice and friendly. The last thing I wanted to do was to create a scene by demonstrating my dissatisfaction with their poor compliance with my advice. I avoided looking at the couple and looked instead at their baby, and in a low but emphatic tone I asked both of the parents why Andrew had not yet been examined by the urologist.

A silence fell on the room, broken only by the smacking sounds Andrew made while savoring his bottle of formula. I heard a subdued whisper: the spouses were eagerly discussing something between themselves. All I could hear was Melody's repeated appeal to her husband, "Show him, show him!" Before I had figured out how to interpret these strange words, I heard the deep, manly voice of Mr. McDonald say, with embarrassment, "Doc, should we really worry about this problem?" Hesitantly, he continued, "Maybe this is just one of those things that run in the family?"

"Anything can run in the family," I answered thoughtfully, "but how are we going to prove it?"

Then it dawned on me.

"Do you mean, Mr. McDonald," I said, "that your, if I may say so, private part, has the same characteristic as your son's, sir?"

"Yes, Doc, exactly so," Stanley answered cheerfully and with a noticeable feeling of relief. "You are exactly right."

"Shall we see it?" I offered, looking straight at Mr. McDonald, who, so it seemed to me, had been waiting for this moment to come.

In an instant he opened the zipper of his jeans, stuck his hand in his fly, and without further delay fished out the organ that had been an invaluable part of Andrew's conception.

Mr. McDonald's private part was in proportion with the large dimensions of his body. When Mr. McDonald took his hand away and let it go, it immediately took exactly the same position as his child's, with its head rotated to face the left thigh.

Giving one more look at this subject of much attentive scrutiny, I indicated that I was fully satisfied with the results of the examination.

While Stanley was quickly closing the zipper of his jeans, I asked him about his experience with having such an unusual physiological deviation. With great conviction he reassured me that everything was fine with both his and Andrew's male organs.

"Well," I said, "it's clear to me now that you are perfectly satisfied with the small anatomical problem that runs in your family."

"Doc, we don't mind. We like it this way," Stanley said in a trusting manner.

I understood that I should never again recommend to the

McDonalds that they take little Andrew in for a consultation with a urologist. I have respected their prudent opinion that Nature has its own ways—ways that doctors sometimes cannot fathom.

This case happened fourteen years ago; since then I have observed similar manifestations of healthy variation of human anatomy on two more occasions, but, after the lesson I learned from the McDonalds, I was not too quick to refer these patients to a specialist.

ON A DARE

NINE YEARS ago, the first child of Debbie and Chad Grisham died in her sleep of sudden infant death syndrome. Two years later, Debbie delivered a strong and healthy daughter at Doctors' Community Hospital. I first met them after the birth of this child, when I was chosen to be the baby's pediatrician.

The memory of the dramatic loss of their first child haunted both parents and transformed any innocent sneeze or cough of their newborn baby into a major event. These anxieties did not prevent their newborn baby, Lana, from being discharged in good condition from the hospital when she was three days old.

Four months later, Lana was admitted to the same hospital for treatment of bronchiolitis, a condition that is not usually serious enough to require hospitalization. Unfortunately, Lana was coughing and wheezing, she had a high respiration rate and significant fever, and therefore she needed to be monitored and treated.

A description of the tense mental condition of both parents during this period of time would take many pages. I was doing my best to reassure them that the outcome of bronchiolitis is usually good, but the unhealed trauma of the Grishams' earlier loss prevented them from thinking rationally.

Lana, who did not share in these parental worries, received appropriate treatment for her condition, and was sent home after three days in the hospital.

Everything passes, and time heals even the worst wounds. The Grishams were able to overcome the despair they felt over the loss of their first child, while Lana grew up successfully, to the joy of her parents.

Two years later, the Grishams had another addition to their family. Baby Farrah was born at the same hospital as her older sister. At this time the Grishams were far less anxious and worried than they had been when Lana was born. Like her sister, Farrah was growing up without any serious medical problems. The number of office visits for Farrah's illnesses was half what it had been for Lana.

On one visit Debbie came with Lana, who was now seven, and five-year-old Farrah, both of them nice, pleasant children. Farrah had an earache; her sister had just come along for a visit. They were both tall, well-built children in good general health.

Several years earlier, when Debbie had finally recovered from her tragedy, I discovered that she had a good sense of humor. Since then, whenever she came in with the children, we regularly exchanged a couple of jokes together.

After Farrah's examination, I confirmed Debbie's impression— Farrah had streptococcal tonsillitis. While writing a prescription, I remarked to Debbie that Farrah, for all her bright and alert looks, was an introverted child. Indeed, during the visit she had not uttered a word; her face did her talking for her. She was somehow able to transmit her thoughts with her expressive eyes.

Noticing small bruises on Farrah's legs, I asked Farrah whether she and Lana were good friends. Introverted Farrah was predictably slow in answering.

"Okay friends," Debbie answered for her. "They usually play well together, though sometimes, despite all her smartness, Lana takes advantage of her. Three days ago, for example, she ate horseradish mixed with mustard because of her!"

"Horseradish and mustard? This is definitely something new and different!"

"Well, Lana and her close friend were daring each other to eat horseradish mixed with mustard. Farrah was playing in the backyard, and Lana got hold of her and persuaded her to eat this combination instead of eating it herself." Mrs. Grisham told me this in a tone of voice that implied that eating horseradish blended with mustard recently had become a common pastime among children.

"Farrah, you really look very sharp. Did your sister actually make you eat horseradish and mustard?" I asked her. She remained silent, wearing an impenetrable smile on her face.

Mrs. Grisham explained to me that it had actually been easy for

Lana. According to Farrah, Lana—like Tom Sawyer, who convinced his friends that whitewashing a fence would be fun, had convinced her with such phrases as, "Farrah try it. Ooh, it's so g-r-r-r-eat. It's so c-o-o-o-l."

I still refused to believe that Farrah could be so easily manipulated into such a foolish thing as eating spicy condiments. Lana, who had sat silently in her chair until this moment, decided to confess. "We added ketchup to the horseradish and mustard to make it sweet," she said, blushing profusely.

"Aha!" I exclaimed. "Do you realize, Lana, that you could have made your sister really sick?"

Lana looked at her sister, silently imploring her to interfere.

"I did not eat too much," Farrah finally spoke out, "I ate just a little. I tossed the rest out, so they wouldn't see."

"No, Farrah, you ate too much of that garbage!" interjected her mother. "Now, Doctor, I'd like to know how dangerous it is." "She puked three times and had two episodes of diarrhea."

"Since your daughter ate horseradish and mustard four days ago, Debbie, nothing should happen at this point," I explained to Mrs. Grisham as we left the room.

At the door I distinctly heard Farrah hissing to her sister, "You still owe me a dollar."

6

LIVING TOGETHER

Belonging to a people who historically have been the victims of prejudice, I do my best to be unprejudiced myself and to judge people for what they are. Over my years of pediatric practice the patients whose trust I have held have been members of all religions, creeds, and races.

The composition of the patients at my present office mainly reflects the demography of the area where my office is located. I see children of Afro-American, Irish, Italian, German, Polish, Russian, and Spanish descent, to name a few.

People of all skin colors coexist in harmony at this office and give me a feeling of human unity. Perhaps because my present partner and I were ourselves the victims of racism, it is easier for us to be sensitive to the feelings of people of different ethnic origins and, thus, with the help of the other members of our staff, to achieve this atmosphere of trust and respect. The secret for deserving this trust is very simple: all that is necessary is to treat our neighbors as we would wish to be treated ourselves, to follow the Golden Rule of Judeo-Christian faith. An outstretched hand and a friendly smile mean more than a thousand words.

Despite this good environment it would be unrealistic to expect that all of the old prejudices and hatreds that are still lurking around would not manifest themselves in our office as well. The stories that I present here cover some of my experiences with racism in my office, but they represent an extremely small number of my experiences in my practice. This illustrates how basically healthy and happy are the relationships that I have had an opportunity to observe during my practice.

ONE LESS BIGOT

ONE OF the realities of pediatric practice is that the workload varies and can go from one extreme to the other. There is a general tendency for pediatricians to be busier during the winter months and during the season of school checkups; the number of visits to a pediatric office, however, also depends on things such as epidemics in the community, the exact timing of which cannot be predicted.

While a visit for well-baby care can be scheduled to the mutual satisfaction of both the family and the office, a visit for a sick child cannot be put off for days—an acutely sick child must be seen immediately. These unexpected factors, plus numerous phone calls, plus patients in the hospital, especially those admitted to the emergency room who require monitoring from the office—all create the likelihood that patients might, sometimes, spend an unusually long time waiting to see me, sometimes, an hour or more.

We doctors and the rest of the staff feel bad when a patient's appointment time is inadvertently delayed and do our best to move the patients along quickly, but we are limited in the capacity to solve the problem: those who have already waited for a long time deserve to be examined and treated as carefully as anyone else. Fortunately, most patients, especially the established ones, are well aware of the goodwill that exists on the part of the office personnel and are kind enough to wait patiently for their turn to be examined.

On one of those really hectic days when I was trying, unsuccessfully, to outrun the clock—racing from one exam room to another, listening to complaints, asking questions, examining, prescribing, giving advice, worrying, answering phone calls—in one of the exam rooms I found Harold Hill with his wife, Alma. All of their children—two daughters and a son—had been brought in for symptoms that indicated streptococcal tonsillitis.

Harold operated a laundromat business.

Both he and his wife belonged to the small group of patients who could be characterized as demanding. Though they did not always keep their scheduled appointments, they frequently came to the office without any appointment at all; they demanded unnecessary medications that they "knew" to be better for their children than those I had prescribed; and, despite all this, they were not too enthusiastic or quick in the payment of their bills.

Both Harold and Alma were on the attack in any conversation, always finding something caustic and smart to say. These remarks were never overtly offensive; for many years during our relationship whenever I tried to expose an element of aggression in these remarks, I immediately saw reassuring smiles on their faces, as if the remark was nothing more than a friendly, innocent joke.

My experience with the family told me that I would inevitably get a rebuke for their long wait in my office. I started to work knowing that the moment would come. Surprisingly, it did not materialize. The Hills asked relevant questions and listened attentively to my advice. They have probably learned their lesson, I thought to myself, after I warned them that I did not want to hear any more rude, biting remarks from them.

When the visit was over, I apologized for their long wait and expressed my appreciation for their understanding.

"What a hot day," I exclaimed as I was about to leave. "I feel like I am working in the tropics."

Mr. Hill looked at me with a long, serious face.

"It's not that hot, Doc," he told me in a didactic tone with a discernible note of friendly irony. "You're just trying to do your job quickly, which is good. But Doc," continued Mr. Hill, lowering the tone of his voice, "your waiting room, indeed, looks like we're in the tropics. It looks more and more as if it were in Africa."

The expression on my face must have changed noticeably because Harold stopped abruptly and just looked at me.

"Mr. Hill," I said, "do you realize that this time you have crossed the line?"

"I understand you, Doc," Mr. Hill said with a conciliatory tone. "Sorry, I didn't mean to interfere with your business." Then, trying to make a joke out of it all, he added cynically, "After all, dollar bills are always green no matter who pays them."

"No, you're wrong," I answered. "Everything matters. In fact, I don't want your green dollars for this visit. Instead, would you please look for another pediatrician whose office would not remind you of Africa. I don't think that my office environment is good enough for you. In the meantime, for the next month I will provide only emergency services for your children." I left the room.

AGAINST THE HAIR

EACH CHILD is different and unique. In each child I see features that belong to one, and only to one, human being. These features distinguish the child from other people and help make that child an individual. The external differences in people help them feel their individuality, preventing them from merging with the nameless crowd, and help them see their special mission in life.

This honest assumption on my part found no support--quite the opposite, in fact—on the part of Monica Foster, who had accompanied her four-year-old, Terence, for a visit to the office. Mrs. Foster worked as a social worker for some agency. We had never had any conflicts during the two years of our acquaintance.

Terence had a small problem: he had developed a rash on his neck and on the scalp area, which had lasted for a week.

After carefully examining his scalp lesions, I turned my attention to Terence's hair. It did not look unusual, but, maybe because it was cut so short, it was firm and resilient. It stuck out like a million little springs on his head.

"Terence, your hair looks like little wires; you can poke your fingers with it," I said with a smile and turned to Mrs. Foster. In place of the reciprocal smile of understanding I had expected, I saw an expression of anger on her face that showed her fierce rejection to what I had said.

"It is none of your business, sir," she said in a harsh and unyielding voice. "You made this disparaging racial remark because he is a black child."

I felt as if she were whipping me with her words. I was hurt by this completely undeserved rebuff: I would have uttered the same remark to a child of any race if I had encountered on his head such special hair as her son had. Besides, I knew that the appearance of Terence's hair could be either a familial characteristic or the sign of a rare condition. Mrs. Foster, however, had a preconceived notion of me. I realized that I would need her goodwill if I was to persuade her to listen to my explanation of why her words were without justification. Unfortunately, Mrs. Foster did not demonstrate this goodwill.

"Just keep working," she said to me abruptly as I tried to object to her words.

"I will not continue working," I protested, choking with emotion, "if you do not let me tell you what I think of your insulting remark." Mrs. Foster was silent.

"I was the subject of bigoted hatred every day of my life from the time I was born until I came to this country when I was thirty. Do not tell me about prejudice—I would be the last one to have it. I have fought against prejudice all my life. Do you understand what I am saying?"

There was no answer from Mrs. Foster.

I finished the examination in silence, stroking Terence's round head with my hand. I knew that I would never see him in my office again.

Mrs. Foster remained silent when I told her that some congenital conditions might cause hair to look like Terence's and advised her to have a consultation with a dermatologist; I then handed her a prescription and left the exam room.

A dark abyss of misunderstanding lay between us.

ADDING INSULT TO INJURY

"YOU LOOK familiar to me. Have we met before?" It seemed to me that both my partner, Michael Nisengolts, and I were using this routine out of force of habit much more frequently than was justified. One morning when we had a new family that had come into our office for the first time, and he made this comment to them, I mentioned this to Michael, but he reassured me that it was nothing to worry about.

Later, during the second session of the same working day, we had another new family in the office. Referred by one of our old patients, Timothy and Paula Shedd were a nice looking, well-dressed, middle-class black couple who had come in for a "get acquainted" visit with us along with their three wonderful children. The children—all of them girls—had pleasant appearances and good manners like their parents.

After the initial introduction I looked at Mr. Shedd and really had the impression that his face looked familiar to me. I tried to remember who he reminded me of. Only two days later, while watching television, did I realize that Mr. Shedd had reminded me of my favorite actor, Bill Cosby.

Meanwhile, after staring at Mr. Shedd's face for some time, I finally told him of the difficulty I was having in figuring out who he looked like to me.

Mr. Shedd must have had a hard day at work before he came into the office. With a smirk on his face, he retorted, "All blacks look alike. Right, Doctor?"

I gave him a radiant smile in response, though inside I felt as if a great wave had hit me.

"Sir, you're wrong in your suspicions," I told him. "More than half of this pediatric practice consists of black patients. Do you think that those people are so unintelligent that they would come to a place if they were not treated with respect and honor?"

To my relief my argument convinced Mr. Shedd. Not only did he back off, but he gave me more opportunities to dispel his unfounded distrust.

While we were talking, I heard my partner's voice coming from the corridor. I opened the door and invited him to meet our potential patients. He entered the room with a hospitable and welcoming smile on his face.

Habit is second nature. He introduced himself to the family and then, looking at Mrs. Shedd, asked her in a good-natured way, "You look very familiar to me. Have I met you before?"

A silent scene followed in which I would rather not have been present. I closed my eyes as I nervously awaited an emotional outburst from the Shedds. A moment passed, and then another, but nothing ensued.

Without delay, I began to try to defuse the explosive situation. Meanwhile, poor Michael looked at me in confusion, trying to understand the reason for my unusual bustling and busy attitude.

Though we parted peacefully, I was afraid that the similarity of Michael's and my innocent remarks might make my reassurance to the Shedds sound unconvincing.

Fortunately, my fears were unfounded. I was pleased to discover that on their way out of the office the Shedds had scheduled an appointment for their children for the next week. Later, their children became our established patients.

GOD WITH A HEART AFFLICTED ME

ON TUESDAYS the office is open late to accommodate working parents. On one of these late evenings I entered the examining room to perform a checkup on an eighteen-month-old infant, Martina Watkins-Malon. Her parents, Darius Watkins and Tanara Malon, were both in the room with her.

Before I could begin to take a history from the family Ms. Malon, a woman in her early thirties with a pleasant, kind face and a graceful way of moving, apologized and asked if I would excuse her for a moment—she needed to change her child's diaper and wanted to do this in the washroom.

I was left in the exam room with Mr. Watkins. Dressed in a brightly colored T-shirt, he sat opposite me, leaning his elbows on the desk and answering my questions. Mr. Watkins, who was in his midthirties, worked as a plumber. He was not tall and had regular, stern facial features. It was obvious that Mr. Watkins was a serious man.

His outer appearance betrayed his desire to make himself look distinct from other people: his haircut was very elaborate, with intricate, zigzagged lines on both sides of his head; his small ears were pierced, and in each ear he wore four gold earring studs set with precious stones. The colors were symmetrically matched on both sides.

Mr. Watkins answered my questions diligently. When I asked him the name of his daughter's previous physician, he took his elbows off the desk, put his hand into the pocket of his trousers for his wallet, and then retrieved the business card of the pediatrician from it. At that moment something clicked with me. I noticed the printing on his T-shirt: the word "FARRAKHAN" was printed across his chest in large italic letters.

Before Mr. Watkins could hand the business card to me I made a sign with my hand for him to wait.

"Mr. Watkins," I said, "I just noticed the 'Farrakhan' written across your T-shirt. Does this mean that Mr. Louis Farrakhan is your spiritual leader?"

Mr. Watkins thought for a moment and nodded, confirming my question.

"In that case, Mr. Watkins, and with all due respect to you and to your child, I feel it would be better for your own sake if you found another pediatrician before our relations become established. The fact of the matter is, Mr. Watkins, that I am Jewish. I came from Russia almost twenty years ago. In Russia I lost nearly every member of my extended family to the atrocities committed by the German executioners whose spiritual leader was Adolf Hitler.

"Your spiritual leader, Mr. Farrakhan, states that the religion of my fathers is the religion of the gutter. Like Hitler he accuses the Jews of all the evil in the world, and, like Hitler, he passionately hates the Jews. Mr. Farrakhan has also claimed to find positive points in Hitler's ideology.

"I do not want to change your ideology, Mr. Watkins. Not at all. I just think you might not want to have a pediatrician for your child who is a Jew.

"For my part, I would expect that you would distrust me. Not only am I a doctor, but I am a human as well, and your presence would create stress for me that could interfere with my providing quality medical care to your child.

"Thus, I really think, Mr. Watkins, that it would be to our mutual benefit if you were to find another pediatrician. There are plenty of good pediatricians around."

I finished this statement, and waited for Mr. Watkins to respond.

Not a muscle on his face moved. He was not looking at me, but I knew that he had heard what I said. I knew that this conversation was tricky and unpredictable and could turn ugly. but I did not regret my words. They were hard for me to speak, but no one could have said them in my stead. To keep silent would have caused me to lose my self-respect—I needed to speak out.

Finally Mr. Watkins turned to me and said in a low, quiet, peaceful voice, "I understand what you are saying about Farrakhan, but I recently read a letter in which he had changed some of his views about Jewish people."

He stopped and then concluded, "I don't want to go to another office. I like this one."

"I did not hear that Mr. Farrakhan had retracted his statements, Mr. Watkins," I remarked.

Before I could finish this thought, the door of the office opened, and Ms. Malon entered, carrying a washed and freshly dressed Martina.

After she entered the room, she passed the baby to Mr. Watkins. At that moment it appeared that Mr. Watkins had completely forgotten about our conversation. He took his daughter and kissed her affectionately. To my surprise the child did not respond with the reaction of a normal baby—she only smiled a wide, happy smile, but did not utter a sound.

I looked more carefully and noticed that the size of Martina's head was much smaller than would be expected for a baby of her age and size.

I realized that Martina had pronounced microcephaly—her head, and thus her brain, was small and underdeveloped. This eighteen-month-old child was functioning at about the level of a four-month-old. The prognosis for such severe microcephaly was very poor, the child was destined to be tremendously mentally disabled.

"I did not know that your child had a problem," I said. "Did your doctor tell you why Martina was born microcephalic?"

"Oh, Doctor, you noticed it," said Ms. Malon with unexpected gratitude. A slight smile appeared on her face. "Yes, she was born like that because when I was pregnant, I had a toxoplasmosis infection. Next time I come I will bring you Martina's medical records. I put them on the dresser to bring them and then forgot."

"What did your doctor tell you about Martina's outlook," I asked Ms. Malon while Mr. Watkins was talking and smiling to his child. Though Martina was smiling back to him with a senseless smile and a vacuous stare, Mr. Watkins appeared to be really enjoying communication with his daughter. Martina was as dear and close to him as if she were a healthy child.

"They told me," answered Ms. Malon, "that she might have serious handicaps in the future."

"She will not," interjected Mr. Watkins, this time in a loud voice. "She's going to be fine. Look, Tanara, didn't you tell me that recently she started to say 'ma-ma.' Just wait and see.

"Right, Martina, baby?" he said to his daughter.

I felt the anger that I had experienced only a moment before melt away. How could I apply the regular criteria of good and evil to Mr. Watkins, given the irremediable affliction of his poor child?

My suffering was in the past and, hopefully, would not be in the future; if his suffering was not right now in the present, then certainly it would be in his future.

I thought that if Mr. Watkins was able to demonstrate such noble human qualities as compassion, devotion, and love for this child, then at some critical moment of history he would be able to make the right choice between good and evil.

Three years later Martina is still my patient. She remains severely handicapped. Her father and mother still come to my office and often demonstrate their inexhaustible love for their daughter. I have never seen Mr. Watkins in his Farrakhan t-shirt again.

AN UNANNOUNCED VISIT

ONCE, AT the end of the day, I discovered several sheets of paper, stapled together, that a parent of one of my patients had left in the examining room. My medical assistant was ready to toss these papers away when I asked her to give them to me. As I scanned the pages, I soon realized that they contained a rabidly racist article, filled with the kind of insane accusations that had been familiar to me from an early age. Attached to the back of these papers was an envelope from which I could clearly see that the package belonged to a family that I knew quite well.

Two-year-old Tammy Saxton and her mother, Ava Saxton, were frequent visitors to my office, as Tammy was predisposed to frequent bronchial asthma attacks. Indeed, when she was twenty months old, Tammy had developed a serious bronchial asthma after a viral infection. Because of shortness of breath, poor air exchange, and low oxygen saturation in her blood, she needed to be hospitalized immediately in a specialized pediatric care unit. Tammy was running a high fever, was constantly coughing, crying, and looked very sick.

Her mother was very upset and, or so it seemed to me, angry. She sat on the examining table, pressing Tammy tightly to her body so that Tammy's head was buried against her chest. She was staring into space and, in a loud and demanding voice, repeated again and again the cliché that was familiar to me: "I cannot understand why my daughter is so sick!" In my experience such a statement invariably is meant as an indirect reproach to the physician for the perceived inappropriate management of the patient's health condition.

I could have told Mrs. Saxton, that bronchial asthma cannot always be well controlled despite the best possible efforts, but I decided to leave this explanation for the future. The child was acutely sick: that was the main priority.

As quickly as possible, Tammy was conveyed via a specialized ambulance to a university hospital. She was discharged in three days, and after that was frequently examined in our office until she had completely recovered. After Tammy's discharge, I did not have any desire to remind Mrs. Saxton of her aggressive outburst; our discussions were limited to professional matters.

When I was reading the venomous material Mrs. Saxton had left behind, my first thought was that she had left it as a personal message, but I immediately realized that since her name was on the envelope, this suspicion should be ruled out.

I read the article again to convince myself that the paper really contained the kind of hateful propaganda I had assumed. In twelve pages a person who called himself a minister viciously attacked Jews and generously praised Hitler for his policies toward them. He also vented lot of spleen against the anti-Castro Cubans and against Asians, and made some racial remarks about whites in general as well.

I informed a civil rights organization about the incident, and it began an investigation. The next measure I took was to inform the family that this kind of hateful propaganda was not compatible with our future relations. After thoroughly analyzing the situation, I decided to do this by sending a letter, enclosing a copy of the article, to the Saxtons' insurance company. I asked the insurance company to help the Saxtons find another pediatrician.

My happiness in being a citizen of the United States filled my consciousness. In the former Soviet Union, complaining about such a matter to any organization would have been a ridiculous waste of time. Though I was not born in the United States, I have more civil rights here than I would ever have had in the former Soviet Union, which used to claim to be an embodiment of socialist internationalism. The materials left in my office reminded me of the many years of humiliation, prejudice, anger, and hate that I had both observed and experienced in the old country.

Though I realized that I lived within the safety of a real democracy, where the rights of each individual are respected, my recollections of this carrier of bigotry, Mrs. Saxton, disturbed my peace of mind. To banish the incident, I immersed myself in my work and tried to forget about it. I had lived and worked in the United States long enough to know that this ugly event was an exception to the rule. Racial or cultural intolerance was something I rarely witnessed in my busy office.

Two weeks later, a representative of the Saxtons' insurance company, an Afro-American woman, called me during office hours. She let me know in no uncertain terms that she understood and shared my anger and outrage at the remarks made in the article. Beginning the following month, she informed me, the Saxtons would be requested to choose another pediatrician for their daughter. My heart filled with joy—once again I had the chance to see American justice and democracy in action.

Another week passed. At the end of a long evening and despite our best efforts, we still had many patients to see. While I was examining a patient, a receptionist asked me to step out. In an anxious tone, she told me that the Saxtons—father, mother, and daughter—had all come to the office without an appointment. The receptionist told me that Mr. Saxton was very nervous, practically shaking and demanded to see me immediately.

With an office full of children and in the middle of a thousand things I still had to do, an unscheduled appointment with the Saxton family did not seem like a great idea at all. Moreover, if the article I found did reflect the attitudes of the Saxtons, the encounter might even turn violent. I wanted neither violence nor a minisymposium on racial issues to occur in my office during this busy time—or at any time, for that matter.

Someone offered to call the police, but I really wanted a peaceful and quiet solution to the problem without outside intervention. After all, I had not initiated the conflict, and my friends were around me. Besides, we needed to settle this issue once and for all.

I asked the receptionist to invite the Saxtons into my office. I was sitting at my desk when Mr. Saxton came in, followed by his wife and daughter. They both held Tammy's hand.

Mr. Saxton was visibly excited, his eyes were sparkling, and his face was very tense and nervous, while Mrs. Saxton's face, which was very familiar to me, was only slightly anxious. She avoided making eye contact with me.

Before they could sit down, little Tammy loosened her hand from her parents and ran toward my desk. To Tammy, I did not look different from other people—children do not divide humanity by race. She recognized me and, eschewing any unnecessary formalities, stretched out her little hand to me and pronounced one word: "Candy!"

At this moment I felt the tension leave me. Tammy belonged to a world that I could understand, a world of trustful, sharing human relations. Her parents should not have been any different from her. I gave Tammy her piece of candy and turned toward Mr. Saxton, waiting for him to start the conversation.

"An insurance company rep called my wife's office. They told her that you had requested that we find another pediatrician. Was that your idea?" asked Mr. Saxton.

"Yes, it was my idea," I confirmed. "Did the representative of your insurance company tell you the reason for my request? Are you aware of the racist, propagandistic article your wife left behind in my office during the last visit?"

"Yes, my wife told me that she forgot some papers at your office," replied Mr. Saxton, his voice becoming more tense, "and this is why we took off time from our jobs to come here. On the way over we picked up our daughter from the baby-sitter."

A silence fell. I wondered what would happen next.

By now, Mr. Saxton appeared highly charged; his voice cracked with tension. After a pause, he continued: "We came to your office to apologize. Neither of us had read that article, and we want you to know that we do not share or support the racist opinions expressed there. I believe that all people should be respected equally, regardless of their race, the color of skin, or their religion. Neither Ava or I have ever had anything to do with this kind of propaganda!"

I turned toward his wife. "Mrs. Saxton, do you really agree with your husband's statement?"

Mrs. Saxton was not as eloquent as her husband in her response. In two short sentences she repeated the apology and also said that she did not agree with the ideas in the article.

"How do you explain the fact that this material was in your possession?" I asked.

"An acquaintance told me a while ago that she wanted to send me the information that might be of interest to me. I had received the envelope at the end of the day when I came to your office. I grabbed the papers, picked up Tammy, and came to your office for her appointment. I did not have any idea what was in the article because I had not yet read a line of it."

She spoke earnestly, sincerely, and spontaneously and strongly persuaded me of her honesty.

I knew that, because of the nature of the conflict, the Saxtons were under no obligation to give me any apology. The insurance company was not a civil rights organization and would have found them another pediatrician without any unpleasant consequences for the family. The Saxtons had come to my office for only one reason: to apologize and to assuage their and my feelings.

A wave of emotion surged inside me. Despite my initial firm resolution not to discuss this matter on a personal level, the words came out of my mouth by themselves. As briefly as I could, both because patients were waiting for me and because I did not want to be misinterpreted, I told the Saxtons about the terrible time my extended family had gone through during World War II as a result of prejudice and racist propaganda.

How could I express in such a limited time my life experience with anti-Semitism? I tried not to open the deep wells of memory; they were still full of the day-to-day episodes of irrational prejudice, hate, and anger that I had observed during the first three decades of my life.

While my voice remained firm and steady, unwelcome tears began filling my eyes, blurring the people and things around me. I told the Saxtons how sad it made me feel that people should divide themselves into groups, cultivate prejudice against each other, and decide that they should be able to select who should be permitted to be born or to live and who should be eliminated.

"I have tried to live in an environment free of the prejudices that surrounded me for so many years. If there is still a degree of distrust between you and anybody who works in this office, all I ask is that you speak neither words of false praise nor words of hatred. All I want," I concluded in a now choked voice, "is just to be left alone. Just to be left alone."

"Doctor, what else can we say?" replied Mr. Saxton. "In what other words could we express our sorrow and regret? We have also come to ask you to keep our daughter under your care."

"You are right," I said. "If I do not believe you, then who will I believe?"

I was overwhelmed. Only twenty years before, I had been just another refugee to this country who, with only a few pieces of luggage, came with my wife and son to flee from persecution and intolerance. Now, two citizens of this country, Ava and Walter Saxton, who, unlike me, had both been born here, had come to me, another citizen, to express our equality and thus demonstrate their sensitivity to my feelings and their own natural decency and integrity.

"Mr. and Mrs. Saxton," I said, "this office fully accepts your apology. I firmly believe that it is sincere and genuine. Please, call your insurance company and tell them that we would be privileged to continue to have your daughter as our patient."

I exchanged firm handshakes with the Saxtons.

Peace and harmony were reestablished in the office. If what had happened here was possible, it gave me hope. The sounds of Beethoven's Ninth Symphony reverberated inside my head.

At this moment, I felt some small, sticky fingers touching my hand. Tammy was looking at me with penetrating, demanding eyes. She was asking for another piece of candy.

A HYPERACTIVE CHILD

MY NEW patient, four-year-old Fritz Schauffler had been born in West Germany and had arrived in the United States only a month before. From his record, I learned that Fritz's parents were no longer married. His father's name was Wilhelm and his stepmother's was Melissa. The family was covered by an insurance carrier that covers military personnel. The Schaufflers were both in their mid-twenties; in addition to Fritz they also had two children of their own—a one-year-old daughter, Elsa, and a two-year-old daughter, Erna. The Schauffler family resided in a racially integrated suburb where both blue- and white-collar families lived.

I guessed that Melissa, Wilhelm's new wife, had been serving in the military at a United States base in West Germany when she and Wilhelm met.

I entered the examining room and introduced myself to Mr. Schauffler and his son. After a short interview, I found that my speculation had been correct: indeed, Wilhelm had met his wife at a base in Germany where he had been teaching German in the local military school. Now the family had come to the United States for permanent residence.

Wilhelm's face had the strong, regular features of a man of Germanic descent. His height was above average, and he looked strong, healthy, and self-assured. He was cleanly shaven and was carefully dressed in an expensive athletic suit. A half-century ago, he could have been used by racial theorists as the model of their glorified so-called Aryan race.

Fritz looked nothing like his father. He apparently bore more resemblance to his mother, who was still living in Germany. His eyes were not deep blue like his father's, but were instead dark; his face was round and his hair was not straight, but curly. His skin, however, was as fair as his father's, and they were also similar in that Fritz had his father's strong cleft chin.

Fritz was a healthy boy; he radiated the strength and vitality of a fast-growing organism. He had came to my office to have his medical forms filled out for his new school.

Fritz sat on the examining table waiting impatiently for his checkup and, no doubt, not so impatiently for a vaccination if it was found that he needed one.

He was all in motion with his four extremities jiggling. He frequently blinked his eyes and rubbed them with his hands. Turning his head from side to side he would look in all directions, but at the same time he was not concentrating on any one object for a long period of time. His incessant motion betrayed some of the features of a hyperactive child.

Though Wilhelm spoke with a noticeable German accent, he spoke English very well for a person who had spent less than two months in this country. In the process of our conversation he asked me many questions about my office and about the other doctors who worked in the practice with me. In a short time, we had established a friendly, relaxed conversation.

Wilhelm made a pleasant impression on me. Listening to his accent, I thought of my favorite composers, Bach, Mozart, and Beethoven; my favorite writers, Goethe, Thomas Mann, and Henrik

Böll; and my favorite poets, Schiller, Heinrich Heine, and Rainer Maria Rilke. The works of these great men, all of whom spoke German, had given me many of my ideas of humanism.

It was not out of my need, but for Wilhelm—to prevent him from any "disappointment"—that I decided to let him know more about me.

"Mr. Schauffler," I told him, "I don't know whether you already knew, but I am Jewish. Personally, it absolutely does not matter who I treat—I am a doctor and my responsibility is to help any human being. I'm sure that you share this attitude, but we live in the real world, and, to some people, it might be important to know about their doctor's descent."

In the U.S.S.R., where century-old prejudices are still alive and well, I had gotten used to hearing the patronizing "compliment" made by some well-meaning people—"Vladimir," they would say in a patronizing and approving manner, "though you are a Jew, still you are a good man."

From Wilhelm, who now stood in front of me, I had expected to hear that it did not bother him at all that his son's doctor was a Jew.

I was mistaken. What I heard from Wilhelm was unexpected. It told me something about the new generation of Germans who were sincerely trying to learn from the horrible experience of Nazi Germany.

"As a Jew, you probably do not like Germans," he said to me looking straight into my eyes.

I thought to myself that dislike and hate are destructive, not constructive feelings. I never thought that an entire nation could be held accountable for the crimes and ideology of some of its sick people. All my life, I have wanted not to be judged based on who my parents were but on who I am. I am not the judge of the German people. God is the common judge for the all human race; let Him judge.

"No, Mr. Schauffler, I do not dislike German people. I do not dislike people of any race or nationality as a matter of fact. You should forgive me, but I just thought that it might be important for you to know that a Jew would be treating your children."

"Doctor," Wilhelm said with an ironic smile, "You should not have any suspicions about me. You might not know it, but my present wife is black."

No more was said on the subject. A mutual understanding had been established between us, and I continued with Fritz's physical examination. He took the procedures and vaccinations stoically, without complaints. In a short time, Fritz's school form was ready to be signed.

I exchanged a firm handshake with Wilhelm as he and his son were leaving.

"Doctor, may I ask you one more question about my son?" Wilhelm asked as he turned to go.

"Doctor, you probably noticed that Fritz is overactive," Wilhelm said. When I answered in the affirmative, he went on, "I did not tell you this before, but his mother, my first wife, was a Turkish woman whom I met in Germany. Some of my friends have told me that Fritz does not behave well because his mother is a Turk. Is that true?"

"No," I answered, "he is not overactive because his mother is a Turk. You could have had the same problem if his mother were German or Jewish, for that matter. The child's personality depends on the soul, which he gets from Heaven when he is born. There are no different races in Heaven. There, everybody is equal."

7

THE TOYS ARE THEM— CHILDREN OF DIVORCE

The last three decades of the twentieth century have been characterized by a serious and alarming decline in the American family. One salient indicator of this serious deterioration in the institution of the family is the remarkably high rate of divorce in this country.

Just a decade ago divorced families were in the minority in my practice. Since that time the number of divorces in my area has increased so much that nowadays children in my practice are as likely to grow up in a family headed by a single parent as in an intact nuclear family.

A mountain of research has been dedicated to the damaging effects of divorce on children and parents. It has been established that it takes around three years for adults who have been divorced to regain a sense of stability and order in their life. How much longer must this process of healing take for the children of divorce? Children lack the knowledge, maturity, and psychological preparedness of adults to cope well with the personal catastrophe of separation and abandonment.

Parents, for whom the divorce is a very traumatic experience, frequently forget the plight of their children and let them stew in their own juice of misery and frustration. Not only do children cease to be the first priority for their parents during this trying time, not only are they exposed to the ugly scenes that accompany divorce, but frequently, even at a very young age, they are used by their parents as confidants, advicegivers, and tools to manipulate the other parent.

It's no wonder that, especially in the first two years after a divorce, many children of divorce are subject to tremendous stress and numerous psychosomatic problems, which may leave irreversible changes in their character.

The problems that children have in coping with divorce are many. It is relatively easy to protect children from an infectious disease by inoculating them against it, but there is no way to inoculate a child from the profound psychological influence of divorce. With an infectious disease such symptoms as a rash, fever, or toxic appearance could serve as objective indicators of the child's condition. In a relatively short time, when the cycle of the infectious disease is over, the symptoms subside. In divorce the pain, sorrow, anguish, and guilt that children feel might be invisible to even a close observer, even to the children themselves, and these symptoms do not subside when the divorce is over.

Children can indicate a sore area of their body, but they are unable to realize that it is their soul, their self—the essence of which is not understandable even to mature adults—which is wounded and bleeds.

As is so often the case in many of the social experiments of the modern age, the children are the main casualty. Ask them about the sexual revolution, about feminism, about life-styles, about conventional and nonconventional families—they know nothing about these things. All they want is to have their mother and father around them every day.

And as a former child and as professional who has observed and worked with children most of my adult life, I know definitely that in the heart of a child exists an overwhelming feeling of trust—trust in the goodness, love, and support of those who were directly responsible for bringing him or her to this world; this instinctive human trust then extends to all human beings in general. With a normal upbringing the child retains this healthy, positive attitude toward people, while the child who lives in an environment devoid of human warmth grows up to be suspicious and fearful of people.

Children universally take it for granted that their parents love them and will never abandon them. Especially at a younger age, they do not care that their parents are incompatible. Their deep psychological need for their parents is as natural as any other basic instinct. Not by bread alone—a child needs not only food, water, and shelter but also a loving family to provide these things to him.

Thus, in divorce, when children lose control of their immediate environment, when they feel that their needs have ceased to be the first priority of their parents, when their parents betray their intuitive expectations, children perceive this as a major personal tragedy. Intimate relations based on feelings of unconditional love lose their sacred value for these children.

Instead of the celebration that life should be at this time, the time when a person's inner self is beginning to blossom like a flower, these children become immersed in feelings of anger, resentment, depression, guilt, and the fear of separation.

No amount of psychotherapy can replace the bliss that a child would feel upon the return of a missing parent—the joy of experiencing this parent's touch, kiss, tender love. No therapist, priest, or rabbi could persuade children of divorce that in the name of modern principles and freedoms, they should cooperate and be content when one of their parents packs up his or her belongings, gives them a good-bye kiss, and disappears—first for a week, then for a month, then for years.

No reassurance, no promise, no comfort that a child receives via psychological or religious intervention can achieve a genuine healing of the soul. The child requires the tangible, material presence of both of parents who were responsible for bringing him or her to life on this planet—this planet of people.

Instead of being used as the last resort in the solution of marital conflicts, divorce has in recent times become an immediate solution to a problem that, more often than not, could have been resolved with a mature give-and-take attitude. If the children's interests were truly the first priority in any decision about an irreversible split, many marriages would be saved. It appears that instead of perfecting the art of surviving alone—a new "religion" of modern times—people should try to learn to live together if they want to restore the institution of family.

This statement does not mean that divorce is always a negative thing. It could be salutary for an abused spouse or for abused children and sometimes when there is considerable incompatibility between spouses. I am not against divorce as an occurrence; I am against divorce as a mass movement.

JOANNE CONTIERRES AND HER TWO SONS

ONE MAJOR source of excitement in pediatrics in having the opportunity to observe the growth and development of a human being. The parent, who sees a child every day, cannot fully understand the pediatrician who exclaims, "Your child has changed so much I can hardly recognize him." If a parent can observe the subtle way in which a child blooms and flourishes daily, the pediatrician is impressed more by the dramatic changes that occur over the interval of months or years.

I remembered Mark Norton from when he was five years old. His mother, Joanne Contierres, who always accompanied him, was with him on this day as well. Mark's problem was not serious; he had a sore throat and cough. He was, at this point, a short handsome young man, whose personality combined the attributes of charisma, gentleness, and contentedness.

I remember Mark's passing from one stage of development to the next. He was always a nice looking, intelligent boy. His only problem was that he was short.

His mother, in her midthirties, looked ten years older than her age. She was a moderately overweight woman who, judging by her tight clothes, was unable to believe her true weight.

Mrs. Contierres had always been unconditionally devoted to her two sons. Mark was the child of Joanne's first marriage; Joanne's other son, five-year-old Patrick, was born from a second marriage. Not only did Joanne have a good relationship with both sons, but they, despite more than ten years difference in their age, were very close as well.

Joanne was also short. Until four years earlier she had been a thin woman, but the asthma that she had suffered from since childhood had gotten worse and become resistant to her usual medications. The large doses of cortisone that were then prescribed resulted in a sharp increase in Joanne's weight.

The poor condition of Joanne's health forced her to quit working full-time. Her main source of income was a monthly $450 disability check that she received from the state. During a time when Joanne was in better health, she supplemented this meager sum by working in a store as a saleswoman on an hourly basis. Joanne's poor health did not break her spirit. Whenever someone tried to offer sympathy Joanne would respond that she was happy that things were not as bad as they could be.

Though Joanne's budget was rigidly limited, her children were carefully dressed, well fed, and beautifully groomed. They were also very well behaved, quiet, and polite children who, like their mother, were uncomplaining and content with life. The only question that Mark always asked me at the end of every visit for the last five years was about his height. He usually asked it in a quiet voice, adding that he did not want to be short. By the age of seventeen he had achieved a height of five feet three inches, which did not make him happy.

"You see, Mark, you are within the normal limits," I told him, trying to cheer him up, as I pointed to where his height fell on the growth chart. "There isn't much you can do to alter nature," I continued. "Look at your mother: she is also short. By the way, how tall is your father?"

"I don't know," Mark answered, looking aside. Then, without exhibiting any strong emotions, he turned toward his mother and re-addressed my question to Joanne with one emphatic word, "Ma?"

"He was also short," Joanne replied. "You see, Mark was only two when his father last saw him," she added, as if she were apologizing for her son's lack of knowledge about his disappeared parent.

"What a shame," I remarked in an impassioned tone. "His father has a son many parents would simply dream of having, and he completely ignores him!"

"It's his loss," Joanne said in a quiet but firm voice, while Mark continued to look off dispassionately, showing us his clean-cut profile.

Mrs. Contierres's second marriage lasted for six years and also ended in divorce. Patrick Roldan, the child of this second marriage, was complaining of fatigue, nausea, and poor appetite when he visited my office during the busy pre-Christmas season.

I had met his father, who worked as a computer operator for an insurance company, only once—when Patrick was born.

After the divorce Patrick's father gave no financial support to his ex-wife and thereby gave none to his own child. He visited his young son less and less frequently.

Patrick's complaints were of a psychosomatic nature, possibly due to divorce-related depression. After Patrick left the exam room for a procedure that was to be performed in the office lab, I asked Joanne how frequently Patrick was visited by his father.

"Every now and then," Joanne answered without enthusiasm.

"What do you mean by 'every now and then'?"

"Well, he used to see him every other weekend, but recently, since he got a girlfriend, it has been once a month and now sometimes less than once a month," she explained.

Seeing that I really wanted to know more about the cause of Patrick's symptoms, Joanne became more enlivened; she gave me a burning look, ready to share the pain in her heart.

"Let me tell you a little secret," Joanne whispered to me, though her son was still out of the room. "You know that despite the big difference in their ages my sons are very close. I recently found out that Mark had a friendly talk with Patrick."

Looking intently at me as if to make sure I was a suitable person with whom to share the intimate, bitter secret that hid behind Joanne's generic smile, she finished in a passionate whisper, "Mark asked him, 'What would you like to have for Christmas?' and Patrick answered him, 'I don't want anything for Christmas. All I want is my father back.'"

FOR BETTY'S SAKE

WITH THE proliferation of managed health care in the field of medicine, the insurance industry has not only labeled pediatricians with the new term of PCP, "primary care providers" but also has commissioned them with a new function: gatekeeper. The PCP gatekeeper prevents patients from incurring unjustifiably high expenses for medical services. For example, the gatekeeper prevents patients from receiving unnecessary and expensive laboratory tests and X rays and forbids the use of specialists outside the specific group of physicians to whom the patient has been assigned by the health care plan. This money-saving policy is implemented and supervised by the insurance company's utilization review committee.

This usually heavily enforced policy was not followed in the case of twenty-month-old Betty Falcon. A representative from her insurance company called me one day, requesting that I refer Betty for a consultation with an allergy and immunology specialist not belonging to her group but practicing instead out of the University of Illinois pediatric clinic.

"Mamie Falcon, Betty's mother, feels that the pneumonia and febrile convulsions that Betty recently experienced, as well as her frequent episodes of ear infections, were the result of low resistance," the representative explained when I asked her what had brought about such an unusual request.

"We know that this problem could be taken care of within the organization," the representative continued, "but the thing is that Ms. Falcon's ex-husband died a week ago from an illness of the liver, and now Ms. Falcon insists that her daughter be treated by the foremost specialists available in Chicago. We feel that in such an unfortunate special situation we ought to satisfy her request regardless of the financial considerations."

Physicians, in their "honorable" capacity as gatekeepers, perform their functions by dispensing their referrals the way the pope gives out special dispensations. These referrals permit the patient to move about within the health care system maze. Referral papers become another symbol of the doctor's authority over the patient's needs in the framework of a rationed health industry.

Ms. Falcon, a divorced mother in her early thirties, had been coming to my office ever since her only child, Betty, was born. She was not distinguished by any special qualities that helped her to stand out in my memory from the many other people who use my pediatric services. I could hardly recollect what she looked like until she started to frequent the office to obtain numerous referrals for her daughter.

Despite my repeated reassurances, Ms. Falcon expected to encounter resistance from me in receiving the necessary referral papers for Betty.

"Please, do not worry, Ms. Falcon, you'll get any referral forms that you need," I told her on several occasions. I also told her that within the health organization to which her daughter presently belonged there were many capable specialists who could provide her with good care. Ms. Falcon politely acknowledged my words, but her tense face told me that she was not swayed in her decision to drive all the way into the city to the University of Illinois pediatric clinic to see one of their allergy and immunology specialists. Even for the preoperative laboratory tests that could easily have been performed at the local hospital, Ms. Falcon insisted on using the lab at the University of Illinois.

Eventually, a full workup of Betty's immunological status was performed, and the results were good. Betty's immunity was found to be reassuringly normal. I did not see her and her mother for four months, until Betty was brought in for a day-care center checkup.

A crying child presents a strikingly different image from that of the same child when happy and laughing. In the past, Betty had usually presented a pitiful picture, but with her recovery from pneumonia and serious ear infection, she was now a pleasure to see. She was not the only one to present this new, pleasant look. Her mother had undergone a similar change. She was no longer tense and apprehensive. Instead, there was a beaming smile on her fine-featured, pretty face. Her look was sincere and friendly. She was nicely dressed and wore long, fine, golden earrings.

There were plenty of things to talk about that had occurred since the last time we had seen each other. While Betty played and had a good time, her mother and I talked of the latest news. Somehow, I won Mamie's favor; speaking with her, I felt that I had become a part of her extended family. This allowed me to inquire about her deceased ex-husband.

"Oh, yes, he is not alive anymore. I thought I told you what happened to him. We lived together for almost a year. Then we divorced. We were already separated when Betty was born. A year ago he developed yellow jaundice, so he went to the doctor. To make a long story short, he was admitted to the hospital and was diagnosed as having an alcoholic cirrhosis. His doctor told him to be very careful and not to smoke or drink, but not only did he go right on doing these things, he also continued to do drugs after his discharge. I am sure he would not have died at thirty-two if not for his insane drug addiction.

"It's a pity, if only because of his child," Mamie continued with a sigh after a short pause. "I feel sorry for poor Betty that she no longer has a father," she concluded.

Mamie stroked her daughter's short hair. Betty, bouncing on the examining table like a ball, was producing joyful sounds of good health and well-being.

Mamie paused for a moment as I examined Betty's ears.

"On the other hand," she continued, returning to her train of thought, "maybe it's for the best that her father is dead."

"Why? What would make you say that?" I was astonished by the harshness of her words.

However, I fully understood Mamie's answer. Despite seeming differences between us—indeed, we grew up on different sides of this planet, and in totally different environments—our values were similar. She told me what I would have heard in similar circumstances from many of the ordinary people from the place where I grew up.

"Because," she answered, becoming more emotional, "because, first of all her father totally ignored her. He saw Betty only on two occasions—once when she was born and once when he came to my house to pick up some clothes he had forgotten when he moved out. And, because of the way things have turned out, I can tell Betty truthfully that her father died of natural causes. Thus, fortunately, she will never find out that her father was a drug addict and an alcoholic."

"Good luck to you, Ms. Falcon. With the way you look now, I would not be surprised to hear on your next visit that you had found a nice man to give you and Betty what you both deserve—love and respect," I said at our parting.

"I surely hope so, Doctor," Mamie answered with an optimistic smile on her face, "At least for Betty's sake, I've got to try."

THE GOLDEN RULE

ANNA OKSAMIT was in perfect physical health. She was of average height with a proportionally built body. She dressed conservatively, wearing a suit and lowheeled shoes. Her pleasant but unexpressive face was distinguished by smooth, lustrous skin. Anna had her hands full. Except for the weekends, her daily routine was quite monotonous: in the morning she drove to the bank where she worked as a supervisor. After working a full day, she returned home to take care of her three children: twelve-year-old Reese, eight-year-old Daniella, and six-year-old May. Her children had been coming to my office for two years. They appeared to be happy, well groomed, and nicely dressed.

Anna's husband, Ralph, had lived with her and helped her raise their children for more than ten years. Their marital bliss ended one afternoon when, to her amazement, Anna saw Ralph packing his clothes and personal items into three suitcases.

Anna was never an emotional person. In a calm voice, almost a monotone, she asked Ralph why he was packing. Ralph, who had never argued with his wife, told Anna in a subdued and unexcited tone that he had recently decided to get a separation from her. The reason, he continued, was the irreconcilable difference between their characters—he was "an outgoing man," and she was "all inside." She would never be able to give him, he told her, something that was very important to him but that he was unable to express in words. There was no other woman involved. He still respected Anna a lot. He was going to see their children as frequently as he could.

Anna remained silent; her inability to express herself prevented her from talking.

It appeared that Ralph had intentionally timed his departure for when all the children would be at school. Before closing the last suitcase, he placed a recent picture of each of his three children inside and then added a large, framed family photo that had been taken the Christmas before. Carrying off his suitcases, he did not look back at his wife, who stood motionless against the front door. Ralph left in the Ford Escort they had bought eight years earlier when their second child was born.

When the children came home from school, Anna told them nothing of their father's departure. Later that evening Ralph called home and let each of his children know of his decision, telling them that what he had done was better for him and, eventually, would be best for all of the members of the family. The Oksamits were a close-knit family where the father's word was given trust and respect; the children did not discuss Ralph's decision and, as was expected from them, immediately agreed with him.

The children were unable to believe that their father had left forever—they thought that their parents would soon patch things up. Why not? They had never seen their parents involved in a serious argument before. They expected that soon, some evening, the door would swing open, and they would see their father standing on the threshold, smiling, suitcases in hand. This dream was not coming to pass. Six months had gone by, but he had not returned home.

This did not mean that Ralph did not visit his children. He came to see them and talk with them every weekend and sometimes on weekdays. More frequently than in the past he bought them presents. Together they would go on outings to shopping malls, arcades, the circus, movies, and fast-food restaurants. Anna did not come out to greet Ralph when he came by to pick up the children. She did not want to speak with him, even when, through the children, Ralph asked her to. Anna thought there was nothing to talk about. After all that had happened between her and Ralph, the occasional phone call was more than enough for her.

The family Anna had grown up in was nice and stable, though she could not recall that they ever talked among themselves about their feelings. In her life Anna had followed her father's favorite expression, "Actions speak louder than words." Anna was expressing her dedication to her family through concrete actions: she kept her house in order and her children healthy and provided with food, shelter, and clothing.

In the first years of their marriage, Ralph, who was not very good at self-expression himself, had, on several occasions, asked Anna to talk with him, but Anna never took this request seriously. Eventually Ralph stopped his invitations for conversation. Anna really could not understand why they should speak if everything was clear between them without words. Even more so now, when they no longer lived together, what benefit could she expect from conversation?

Little by little a new pattern became established in the Oksamit family. May and Reese behaved as if nothing had happened. Indeed, even though their father no longer lived with them, he was still living in the neighborhood. Since Ralph worked as a policeman at the local station, he was immediately available not only by phone but in person as well anytime his children needed him.

May and Reese soon became involved in school activities and sports, which kept them occupied. Only Daniella, for some unknown reason, refused to accept the new order. Initially, she participated in the family ritual of silence as well, but she soon began asking and then demanding of her mother an explanation for her father's decision to leave the family. Since Anna could not give her a good answer, her demands became more and more persistent. Daniella did not understand that her mother could not provide her with an explanation of what she could not understand very well herself.

After several unsuccessful attempts to give Daniella a satisfactory answer, Anna gave up. Whenever she tried to speak not of actions, but of feelings, whenever she dug into her heart for an answer, a sharp, burning pain pierced through her chest and her mind and gave her the sensation that she was going to explode into a thousand throbbing fragments.

For her, Ralph's decision was beyond comprehension. Since she had been a child, she had been told to be brave, to smile, and to keep a stiff upper lip. Even if she had been able to explain to Daniella how difficult it was for her to talk about her feelings, she still would have been unable to explain why her father had left. She told Daniella that such things happen in all kinds of families and that she should not feel upset because of it. What else could she tell her? She could give her children her time and energy; she would gladly give them her last morsel of bread or last sip of water, but she was simply unable to explore the world of emotions.

Daniella was not satisfied. She kept bugging Anna for a suitable answer to her question. When she understood that she could not get a meaningful answer from her mother, she started to charge her father with the same demand. Ralph tried at first to answer her from within the same framework of rationalization as Anna had, but this did not satisfy Daniella. Consequently, Ralph tried to turn Daniella's question into a joke, but his daughter did not buy this either. Like a broken record, she kept asking the same question again and again until Ralph told her that he was sick and tired of "all this silly stuff." How was it that Daniella could not understand that whatever was done was done and that there was nothing more to discuss?

Daniella was well dressed and well fed and cared for, but she needed an answer to her burning question. The lack of it created a void inside her, and her inability to fill this void was making her angrier every day.

A week before Anna brought Daniella to my office, she had returned from school almost at the same time of day as she had from work. Anna gave her usual kiss and then asked Daniella how she was doing. "Ok," was the only response she got from her. Anna was surprised: normally her daughter was more talkative.

"What's the matter with you, Daniel?" she asked, stroking her head with one hand as with the other hand she sorted the mail she had just brought in.

Suddenly she felt Daniella roughly remove her hand from her head. Before she realized what was happening, Daniella began to hit her with all the might of her small fists. She jumped at Anna like a bird, uttering high-pitched, unrecognizable primitive sounds.

Anna finished telling this story to me, while Daniella sat in the waiting room watching television. To get more details, I asked her many questions, but she always answered with the minimal number of words and gestures, as if she thought I could comprehend her story just by looking into her amber eyes.

Initially she had tried to deal with her daughter's problems herself, but, in the face of Daniella's escalating aggressiveness, she decided that she needed outside help.

In addition to her repeated attempts to strike her mother, Daniella was having other behavioral problems: on several occasions she had fought with her siblings; she was experimenting with smoking; and she had made some new friends, whom she refused to drop despite her mother's insistence.

It was time for me to speak with Daniella. Anna went outside and returned with her from the waiting room in a moment. Tall for her age and a pretty girl, Daniella sat across from me with a defiant expression. Her impetuous anger and painful resentment were written all over her; her lips were pressed firmly together into a deep frown. The mental tension she had been exposed to over the last months had left an expression of vague anxiety on her young face that was incongruous with her age.

Such a rebellious, self-protective appearance might have been intimidating to a casual observer. Someone who has had experience with this type of patient, however, knows that behind this rebellious smoke screen hides a scared human soul, a person who is desperately trying to find a solution to a severe internal conflict.

For many years I had been extremely interested in finding out just what mental health specialists did to help their difficult patients. What kind of specific questions did they ask them? What were the unusual, special words they used to magically help these patients?

After many years of study I finally realized that the answer to my question was as great and simple as the Golden Rule, which states "Love your neighbor as yourself." By the same token, if someone wants to help a fellow human being in trouble, he or she has only to ask himself a simple question: what words of consolation would I want to hear if I were in this situation?

I looked attentively at Daniella and discerned on her angry face an expression of sadness, insecurity, and pain.

I then closed my eyes and tried to put myself in Daniella's place. She can no longer have her father and mother together at her home—the home where she was born, where she took her first steps, where she spoke her first words, where she first perceived herself to be a separate human being. To her, her father's departure presented a personal catastrophe. What she needed to hear was the convincing assurance that she was still loved by those who were dearest to her.

Our session continued for more than an hour. At the end of this session I told my visitors that each human being is free to make a choice between two opposite modes of living: the way to a fruitful, constructive life and the way of individual destruction and decay. To support my words I picked up a Bible from the bookshelf and read my favorite passage from the book of Deuteronomy, "I have set before thee life and death, the blessing and the curse; therefore choose life, that thou mayest live." I read this verse mostly for Anna's sake, but, to my surprise, eight-year-old Daniella paid much closer attention and had a keener interest in these profound words than did her mother.

A week later the Oksamits came to my office for their second counseling. Like the previous visit, this one lasted for more than an hour. I was pleased to hear from both Mrs. Oksamit and Daniella that there had been a definite improvement in their relationship since the last time we met. Mrs. Oksamit told me that Daniella had been "in better shape"; in her turn Daniella, who had inherited her parents' style of minimal communication, informed me very sincerely that she was "fine." Even before they spoke with me, I could see in Daniella the wonder of good changes in the making. Though an alert and searching look frequently lit up her eyes, the display of anger and resentment on her face had melted away and had been replaced with by a more typical appearance for a child of her age—an appearance of contentment.

At the end of the meeting, after hugging me, Daniella approached her mother and hugged her as well. The second hug was strong and affectionate. Not saying a word, Anna and Daniella were holding each other as if they had met after a long separation. I would not bet on it, but I thought I saw tears in Anna's eyes.

When the session ended, we decided to meet the next week. When the week had passed, Anna called me and in a businesslike and unemotional manner told me that Daniella's conduct had become so much better that she wondered if it would be Ok if she canceled the session.

"My insurance pays for this type of visits, Doctor, so it isn't the money that I'm trying to save. The only reason I want to cancel is because Daniella really is doing much better."

We decided that if she or Daniella ever felt that another session was necessary, they would let me know immediately.

Two weeks later Daniella came to the office, not for another counseling but for a mild respiratory infection. At the end of the visit I inquired both of her and of Anna about their interpersonal relations. Both Anna and Daniella told me that everything was good. They spoke about the past as if they had already forgotten about the two therapy sessions. Following my principle never to intrude in the sphere of emotional health unless invited, or in the case of a life-threatening situation, I went no further.

Five months passed before I saw the Oksamit family again. On this summer day, while walking along the office corridor I met Anna, who, along with Reese and May, was on the way out of the office after her children had been given a school checkup by another physician in my practice.

"How are you, Mrs. Oksamit" I exclaimed to Anna, who was walking between her children to the exit. Anna noticed me and gave me a smile that, on a scale designed for Mrs. Oksamit, could be qualified as "brighter than a thousand suns," but that, for most people, might go completely unnoticed.

Anna and I stepped aside while her children went to wait for her in the reception area.

"I am very glad to see you again, Mrs. Oksamit" I said. "I cannot wait to hear from you how Daniella is doing? Is she Ok? Are you still on good terms?"

"Daniella is doing fine, no problems, Doctor," Anna replied. "These sessions did help her," she added after a brief pause, looking at me intently.

"Did your husband return to the family?"

"No. But he sees the children every weekend," Anna answered in her reserved manner.

I was happy to hear that Daniella was doing well, but it was difficult for me to believe that after only two sessions of intervention such a success was possible. Trying to emphasize to Mrs. Oksamit the importance of my next question, I took her hand as she continued to give me a look of concentration.

"Mrs. Oksamit, I am very happy to hear that Daniella is doing well. I feel privileged to be one of those who participated in an effort to help her. For my professional experience it is tremendously important to hear from you what the particular words were that helped Daniella."

For Anna, everything was very clear. She did not even pause before answering.

"Well, all the things you told her: that she was a good girl; that it was not her fault that her father left us; that both Ralph and I have never stopped caring for her; that her brother and sister and her father and mother, we all need her," Anna stated matter-of-factly, as usual, hardly exhibiting any emotions.

Suddenly Anna paused. Then, in a choked and muted voice that was quite unusual for her, she said, "Also, all the stuff you told her about love."

"What did I tell her about love, Anna?"

"That I love her, and that her father loves her, that her siblings love her, and that you love her too. That this love will last forever and that we will never abandon her." Anna finished and was then ready to join her children, who were impatiently waiting for her.

We shook hands. Anna went to the exit but suddenly turned to me. I saw a sunny smile on her face. "Would you believe," she said to me in a voice loud enough for her children to hear what she was saying, "on Mother's Day Daniella presented me with a huge bouquet of flowers. She drew a beautiful card for me all by herself. I really do not know where this kid found money to buy me those flowers."

A FAMILY

MAXINE RUTANA'S parents were fond of each other and respected each other, but their characters were very different. This difference could have been easily overlooked by an outside observer because both Dolores and Rusty were energetic, outgoing, life-asserting individuals. If Dolores, however, managed to be accurate with her schedule, was careful about her appearance, and maintained order in the family, Rusty was born to be an anarchist. With all the care and love between them, especially during the first years of their marriage, they were still essentially different types of people who lived in two different worlds.

During their visits to the office, they both revealed happy dispositions—joking between themselves and playing with their daughter Maxine, whom they both adored. But I never saw them exchange with each other more than two or three sentences beyond superficial talk.

Both parents were working, and both were trying to do the best they could with their lives, but the distance between their personalities steadily increased, until, finally, after being married for seven years, they divorced.

Rusty moved to another suburb while Dolores continued to live at their old apartment with Maxine, who was at this time about eight years old.

Rusty was welcome to see Maxine any time and almost never missed an opportunity to visit her, especially on weekends. Rusty rarely came, however, at the scheduled time. He did not intend to be late—he just hated to look at his watch. Maxine rarely knew when her father was going to visit or what they were going to do together. They went to sleep late at night and woke up late the next morning. They had a lot of fun, but at the end of these visits Maxine was exhausted and filled with a feeling of dissatisfaction that was difficult for her to put into words.

Two years after the divorce, Dolores mentioned to me that Maxine was having a discipline problem at school. She soon began to display behavior problems at home as well. Dolores caught her stealing small amounts of money, lying, and mysteriously disappearing from home.

At Dolores's request, I had several family counseling sessions with her and Maxine, during which Maxine appeared to be emotionally charged and avoided speaking to me or making eye contact with me.

"I cannot recognize my Maxine; it's just not like her," Dolores told me at the end of one of these sessions after Maxine had left the room at her request.

"She has changed for the worse, and I can only hope she will improve. Two days ago we were talking—actually I was talking and she was listening—and the end of my talk she looked at me and said, 'I know you're right, Mom, I have to improve.'"

She chuckled and added, "Can you imagine? Maxine, completely on her own, promised me that she would be 'a good girl' like in the good old times."

We had already said good-bye to each other when Dolores looked at me with a bright smile on her face and told me that I would soon hear something very interesting from her.

"It's my secret," she answered, smiling mysteriously, when I asked her to tell me what surprise to expect.

Dolores's secret was that she was pregnant. Four months later (her pregnancy was hardly visible until very near the end) my practice was enriched with a new patient—a wonderful baby, Grant Brandt, the son of Dolores and her boyfriend, Flint Brandt.

From the standpoint of character compatibility Flint was a good match for Dolores. He was a nice looking, down-to-earth young man, slightly overweight, a little taller than Dolores, with a mischievous smile.

"So, when is the wedding, you, happy parents?" I asked Dolores, only somewhat as a joke, as I knew her to be a woman with strong moral values.

"Soon, very soon," Dolores answered. "Believe it or not, we simply have not had time to get married. It all happened so fast. When, to our total surprise, we found out that I was pregnant, we immediately bought a house and some furniture and started to buy some clothes for the baby."

"We did everything but get married. That we forgot," she joked, waving her long, delicate hand.

"However, this is on our agenda, believe me," Dolores continued in a serious tone. "You'll be the first on the invitation list," she promised with a pleasant smile.

I asked Dolores about Maxine. How was she doing? What was her reaction to the arrival of this tiny competitor for her mother's attention?

"It looks like I have killed two birds with one stone," she answered. "Not only am I getting a wonderful husband, but Grant's birth has been very beneficial for Maxine."

"She's a really good older sister. She helps Flint and me a lot with caring for the baby. It looks as if life has become meaningful for her. You would not recognize her. Maybe she is doing much better because she is not as bored as she used to be."

The radical change in her family continued to produce a salutary effect on Maxine. Whenever Dolores came in with little Grant, I heard from her that though Maxine's behavior was still not perfect, she had definitely made a lot of improvement. Maxine's father still came to see her as before, but Maxine also felt a strong attachment to her new family. Though she was still a part of the fragmentary, unpredictable world of joint custody which pulled her heart apart she functioned much better in the wholesome, more secure environment of her close nuclear family.

Her mother kept her word. She and Flint were officially married six months after Grant's birth. Maxine was splendid in her role as a bridesmaid during the wedding ceremony.

BREATHTAKING EXPERIENCES

SEVEN-YEAR-OLD Gabriel Boyce, who was accompanied by his father, Hector Boyce, a thirty-year-old blue-collar worker, had a condition that was very familiar to me. As a matter of fact, the diagnosis could be established just by watching my patient. Gabriel was noisily inhaling until his lungs were full to bursting with air, yet no amount of air could seemingly satisfy his craving; as soon as he exhaled, he would begin greedily gulping in air all over again. This reminded me of the time when my son Sasha had a similar condition some twenty years earlier. At that time we—newly arrived immigrants—were living in a public-housing project on the near north side of Chicago.

My wife and I chose to live in this building because we wanted to see for ourselves how the United States' "melting pot" worked. We were rewarded by our decision: we became acquainted with people of different religions, languages, and skin colors, learned a little about their way of life, and enjoyed having an opportunity to live with them in peace and harmony under the same roof.

A year after we moved into the project, we were robbed, and the robber, as we learned much later, was a maintenance man who worked in the building. When we—my wife, my son, and I—returned from a trip to the immigration agency in downtown Chicago, we found that the most valuable of our meager possessions were gone.

Instead of being upset with our misfortune, we scraped together all of our available money, went to the secondhand store, and bought a used television set for seventy-five dollars. Though our new television had a slightly blurred picture and deep scratches on its cabinet, it was a step up from the one that had been stolen: it had a larger screen and was a color set, not a black-and-white one. Thus, thanks to the robbery, we became the proud owners of a big color television—a luxury that we could not have imagined before coming to this country.

On the evening of the second day after the robbery, we had returned to our normal life, and it seemed that our small mishap was behind us, when our son developed an anxiety neurosis. It showed only one symptom—shortness of breath, or "air hunger." He breathed in deeply and sometimes even yawned, looking like a fish out of water, trying to achieve a feeling of satisfaction from the inhaling phase of the act of breathing. Sometimes deep inspiration was followed by the audible expiration. It took several days for his anxiety and tension to finally abate; with no psychological intervention other than friendly reassurance, the symptom went away by itself.

Back in my office, Mr. Boyce said, "For several days Gabriel has had difficulty breathing. He inhales, but apparently he does not feel that he can get enough of it; it's as if he were smothered. He is hungry for oxygen. He works so hard to get enough air in his lungs that he developed chest pain yesterday. Only when he is alone or sleeping does he breathe normally."

As I expected, a meticulous physical examination of Gabriel, revealed nothing abnormal. While I examined Gabriel, he sighed like an old man who carried the weight of the world on his narrow shoulders.

"Your child appears to be essentially healthy," I summarized my impression to Mr. Boyce. "The symptoms of breathlessness are frequently produced by a state of anxiety or, in laymen's terms, because of 'nerves.'"

"That would be very true for Gabriel," confirmed Mr. Boyce, as if he were expecting just this information. "Gabriel is, indeed, going through a rough time. His mother, my ex-wife, left him and his ten-year-old sister with me more than six months ago after she divorced me. I try to spend as much time as I possibly can with them, but I have to work to feed them. When Gabriel is not at school, my mother watches him.

"The problem with his breathing started three days ago when he learned from me that his mother had remarried. I never expected that this news would affect Gabriel so much: he has hardly spoken of her since she left us, and she never calls or comes to see the children.

"He always liked Nintendo games, but he never played them excessively. Yet, ever since our conversation, all he has done is play Nintendo. All day long he sits in front of the TV screen playing and breathing like he is trying to catch air, like he has a suffocating sensation."

At the end of the visit I recommended that Mr. Boyce take a vacation and spend some time with his children, giving them as much attention, warmth, and love as he could. In addition, during the vacation Mr. Boyce should try to ignore Gabriel's alarming breathing and try to divert him to normal, healthy activities.

I next met the Boyces some two weeks later. Gabriel was completely cured of his anxiety-related breathing problems. His father also looked relaxed and rested.

"Doctor, you gave me great advice," he started. "I took the kids to my sister's place for a vacation; she lives in Florida. Gabriel stopped fighting for air on the second day of the vacation, but this was not the only accomplishment. My sister introduced me to a wonderful woman, a single parent like me. Gabriel became very friendly with this lady's son, who is the same age as Gabriel. They were playing like two good pals. This woman and I also liked each other. Doctor, she is really great. Just looking at her is a breathtaking experience. When we parted, she told me that she would soon come for a visit, and then who knows what we will decide. Maybe my children will have a new brother and a new mother one of these days. Who knows?"

With a contagious smile he concluded, "Yes, Doctor, a vacation is good medicine."

IN AND OUT OF BED

OBESITY BELONGS to the category of health conditions that are a source of major frustration and disappointment to the pediatrician who tries to treat them.

If there is even some small possibility for a physician to explain the harm of obesity to an adult patient, for whom the nucleus of the personality is well established, and to motivate that patient by appealing to reason, such an opportunity is truly limited with a pediatric patient.

A child who has been praised since birth for his good appetite simply does not understand all the fuss over his weight. Even in promising cases where there is a chance to motivate a young patient to lose weight, no significant success is possible without the active participation of other family members, and this is especially true for grandparents.

Whenever I discussed the obvious necessity of losing weight and the ways to achieve this goal with ten-year-old Darlene Runyan, my enthusiasm was quickly diminished when I recollected that her grandparents were still under the impression that their grandchild, who weighed 105 pounds and was four foots, seven inches tall, was still on the thin side.

Darlene's mother, Dolly, was an energetic, cooperative, cheerful, and portly woman in her midthirties. She came from Texas and I had sometimes problem to understand her accent. Darlene's father, who had divorced Dolly seven years earlier, had not contacted either Dolly or Darlene for the last five years.

Darlene's animated face and expressive eyes, her lovely hair, and her straight white teeth were offset by the rest of her appearance. Many people accumulate fat on their body selectively, so that the fat leaves some parts of body, such as the face, unchanged in appearance. On Darlene's body, however, the fat layer had accumulated all over, giving her figure the appearance of a big meatball. The deposits of fat on her face had noticeably distorted its features. Her nose, which was large in proportion to the rest of her face, together with her somewhat receding chin, gave her the look of a big, peculiar fish.

Before we started counseling sessions for Darlene's psychological problems, which was a direct reason for the visit, I told Ms. Runyan that although it was realistic to expect that psychological intervention might help Darlene with the sleep-related problems, the night fears, and anxieties that she was experiencing, it was unrealistic to expect that it would substantially change her obesity.

"I know that," Ms. Runyan replied. "We were going to Weight Watchers together. Both of us have learned a good deal there, and now Darlene watches what she eats. Only, when her grandmothers are cooking for her, she loses her head and forgets all about calories and healthy nutrition. Still, Darlene's main problem is not overeating. Her problem is that she's not active enough."

Dolly complained that Darlene avoided playing outside with her friends and preferred to be indoors all day with her grandmother. She would spend the entire day watching television, sleeping, eating, and daydreaming. In a word, Darlene was escaping from life.

Although she was not interested in any particular subject, she was still performing well at school, but she did her work mechanically, without any particular interest in what she was studying.

Ms. Runyan was unhappy with Darlene's lack of interests but had become used to it. The main reason that she had appealed for my help was her daughter's sleeping problem. For the last two years Darlene had night fears, but over the last two month, every single morning Dolly had found Darlene in bed with her; Darlene was slipping in so quietly and surreptitiously in the night that Dolly was always startled to find her there the next morning.

Politely first and then with growing irritation, Ms. Runyan told Darlene to stop sneaking into her bed, but Darlene, with an air of genuine childish innocence, told her mother that she became frightened at night and slipped into her mother's bed without really knowing that she was doing it.

Darlene listened with sincere interest to our conversation during the first session. Despite any psychological problems she may have had, she was outwardly friendly and cooperative. This lasted until she was challenged to talk about herself. Then she retreated into a shell, and an icy wind of internal passivity numbed my numerous endeavors to establish contact with her on a personal level. There was nothing unusual in this: Darlene was in a state of mild depression. It was difficult for her to function because the internal world of her personality was separated from the external one by some invisible barrier that prevented her from being open and spontaneous.

Despite Darlene's reticent behavior during this session, it was not her mother, but Darlene herself, who carefully saw to it that they did not miss their next appointment.

A month passed, and Ms. Runyan told me that Darlene was making definite progress, at least a little. Ms. Runyan was not too stern a taskmaster—she was happy that Darlene was coming to her bed only three times a week as opposed to every night.

Finally, we came to our last session. Darlene was much more open during this session. Before our parting, with a charming smile on her pudgy face, Darlene asked me how long it took to become a medical doctor. She said she wanted to be a surgeon when she grew up.

After that, the Runyanes disappeared from my horizon for more then two years. Then, one day, I entered an exam room and found two visitors there. One of them I easily recognized as Ms. Runyan, dressed in an elegant business suit. She cheerfully greeted me.

Across from her sat a young lady. I knew that Dolly had only one child, so it was only logical for me to assume that this was Darlene, but was this the Darlene I knew? The Darlene I knew was a big "meatball" of a creature with a fishlike face; only someone who had the chance to communicate closely with her could know that under this exterior beat the heart of a sensitive and tender person. Now, instead of a shapeless, swollen, ovoid figure, before me sat a very attractive, tall, vivacious, and friendly girl with no hint of her past fishlike appearance. My visitor gazed at me intently as if she were challenging me to recognize her and to appreciate the magical change that she had undergone physically and mentally since our last meeting.

After another good look, I recognized in this challenger Darlene's smile and Darlene's eyes. She was wearing some familiar rings on her fingers, and on her wrists I noticed the same handwoven "friendship" bracelets that she had worn two years earlier. Darlene had been transformed from a poorly adjusted child into an apple-pie, all-American girl who could easily blend in with a typical group of her peers.

"Did you recognize my daughter," I heard Dolly's voice. "Doesn't she look different than she did the last time you saw her?"

What had helped Darlene to lose so many pounds of excessive weight so dramatically? What had changed her appearance from that of a person who led a molelike existence to one of a bird who soars high in the blue skies?

"Different?" I replied to Dolly's question. "She is not just different. This is a Darlene I can hardly recognize. I am sure that this change did not take place only as a result of four hour-long counseling sessions, and I cannot wait to hear what the cause of this magical change was."

"First of all, Doctor, the sessions did help her, but, you are right, that was not all."

"I'm sure it wasn't because you won a million-dollar lottery ticket?" I tried to joke.

"No, we did not win the lottery, but we won something worth much more than a million," Dolly continued.

At this moment she was interrupted by Darlene's melodic voice. "My mother got remarried eighteen months ago," she said. "We now have a big family: a mother, a father, my two new sisters, a dog, and a kitten."

"So that's what Darlene was missing during the time she was sneaking into your bed—a big family!" I exclaimed.

"Of course," answered Mrs. Sabel, the former Ms. Runyan. "During the time when we were coming in for sessions I was dating the man who later became my husband. It did not take very long for me to realize that he would not only make a good husband but would be a good stepfather for Darlene, as well.

"Please, do not smile, but I was really apprehensive that during our honeymoon I would share my bed not only with my new husband but with Darlene as well. What I had not realized was Darlene's enormous desire to have a normal family. I do not understand this myself, but from the first day of my marriage she never again sneaked into my bed. Besides, she is not bored anymore, as she used to be. She lives a normal, happy life."

GHOSTS, MONSTERS, AND APPARITIONS

EVA RUZICKA was in her early thirties when she had her first and only child, Carson. After a year in an unhappy marriage, she separated from her husband and later divorced him.

Eva was a woman with good manners who was quiet, reserved, respectful, and friendly. She was tall, with pleasant facial features. A little scar on her forehead, a result of a fall in her early childhood, did not adversely affect her appearance. She listened attentively to my explanations and advice, blinking frequently with her long, thick, light-colored eyelashes while taking notes.

Carson whose father had never appeared in my office, had been my patient since his birth and was brought in for examinations more frequently than the average child until he reached two years of age. It was clear to me that Carson's frequent visits were more for his mother's sake than for his own. Eva needed reassurance that her little son was in good health. Parents, by definition, love their children, but Eva handled her son with the care and caution one would take with a piece of precious china.

Carson was a nice looking, well-kept baby. He was usually quiet until he was examined; then his heartrending, high-pitched, shrill cry would reverberate throughout the office. This happened during all of his visits until he grew out of infancy. To protect myself from a headache and hearing loss, I used to place my stethoscope earpieces in my ears with the disc in the closed position even before he started crying.

From a very young age, an individual child's temperament can usually be predicted by simple observation of his or her behavior. Children who have a greater chance of being aggressive when they grow up usually accompany their crying with active fighting—pulling and scratching the examiner's hands with their hands, jerking their legs, and twisting their bodies while crying. Less aggressive children cry without too much fighting and jerking and allow themselves to be examined in a shorter period of time. Carson belonged to the second category of children. Despite his exceptionally noisy behavior, once the exam was over, he would quickly calm down and just cling to his mother for a while.

On a couple of occasions I remarked to Eva that Carson seemed much too dependent on her, and that it was important for Eva to cut the invisible umbilical cord that still connected them in order for Carson to achieve maturity and the autonomy of his personality. My remark did not cause Eva to become defensive or upset. She listened attentively to me, silently nodding her head as if in agreement, but said nothing.

At every major holiday I received a card from Eva. When Carson became three, the cards started to come from him as well. These cards were always delivered in person by Carson, dressed up for these occasions.

At about the same time that Carson stopped being a crybaby, he gradually began to transform himself into a well-adjusted youngster with a warm, agreeable character. His sweet, friendly smile, which reminded me of the mischievous, naughty smile of Mickey Mouse, was always present on his face. Eva had also become less reticent and more relaxed.

I could now place Carson's temperament into the subdivision of nonaggressive children, those whom I call philosophers. During his exams he took the difficult parts of the visit with stoicism, crying only at the most unpleasant moments and patiently waiting until the visit was over.

Carson had an inborn sense of beauty. He started to draw pictures, sing songs and even play the piano at an early age.

For his sixth birthday, Carson came to the office in a dazzling cowboy costume set off with rhinestones and with patent-leather shoes on his little feet. He greeted me with his charming, friendly smile and, in his dignified manner, handed me his new drawing displaying his artistic talent. In turn, on behalf of the office, I sang "Happy Birthday" to him over the office intercom, so everybody would know that it was Carson's birthday. In conclusion I presented him with a toy clown that was dressed in a striped suit.

"Carson," I said to my delightful patient while his mother beamed at him, "when you were small—you cannot remember this, of course—you were such a crybaby that I used to use my stethoscope as earplugs when you began your crying performance. Now, you are my little hero, and I am proud of you. I wish I knew what changed you from a noisy, scared little chicken into such a fine young man," I muttered, not expecting an answer to my rhetorical remark.

"He changed because his father disappeared from his life." To my surprise, I heard Eva explaining this to me. "Until Carson was about two-and-a-half years old," she continued, "his father had unlimited visitation rights. Nobody believed me when I said that these visits were producing an unhealthy effect on Carson until I was able, ultimately, to prove it."

"I never heard anything from you about Carson's father having a damaging influence on his character. What bad effect was that?"

The following conversation took place in Carson's presence. I personally would have preferred that Carson not hear this story, but it was obvious he had heard it many times before.

"When Carson was about a year old, my husband and I decided to separate. We continued to live in the same apartment, using different rooms and different entrances. We thought that in time we would find a way to live together.

"Usually, my ex-husband took Carson to his part of the apartment on weekends, three or four times a month. Over time I began noticing that Carson was returning from these visits acting irritable and scared, but for a long time I was unable to figure out the reason for his strange behavior. Fortunately, as you remember, he started to speak very early. From the incoherent words I heard from him when he returned from my ex-husband, I finally guessed that this man was telling him some kind of pathological garbage about monsters, ghosts, and spirits. I confronted him with these suspicions at once. Instead of putting me at ease, he told me that Carson is a boy and should be taught how not to be afraid of superstitions, and that Carson was as much his child as mine and it was none of my business what he said to Carson when he visited him.

"I consulted a judge, a lawyer, and a child advocate from the Department of Children and Family Services, but this got me nowhere. They all told me that, with all due respect for my concerns, I did not have a case against Carson's father because it was my word against his. Meanwhile, Carson developed a sleep problem: he would wake up in the middle of the night screaming, shaking, and gasping, unable to recognize me. I was simply desperate. All I could think of was how to substantiate my suspicion that his father was screwing up his mind with this morbid monster stuff. I needed to isolate Carson from his father's destructive influence.

"Unable to passively observe my child becoming a victim to his father's abuse—Carson was becoming more and more scared of everything, clinging to me like a vine—I finally decided that enough was enough. My brother, who is a specialist in electronics, helped me to install a recording device in my ex-husband's half of the apartment. The gibberish he was telling his own child made me sick to my stomach. I would never have believed that anyone would have such a sick and morbid imagination, but here was my ex-husband, whom I thought I knew well, telling his own little baby a bunch of hair-raising balderdash about devils, demons, graves, worms, corpses, blood, and violence.

"I gave a tape with three recorded encounters between my ex-husband and Carson to my lawyer. This recording worked like a magic wand. At this point, I came to the realization that we could no longer avoid a divorce.

"Once Carson stopped seeing his father, his behavior changed for the better, but it took almost a year until he was finally rid of all his anxieties. Thanks to my divorce he became a normal child.

"Right, Carson?" concluded Eva, pressing his amazingly cute child to her chest.

This question sounded rhetorical to me, but Carson took it literally. He looked at his mother with shining eyes, affirmatively nodding his little head, and answered with a strong "Yes, mother, you're right."

8

ABANDONMENT OF CHILDREN

Three years ago, on coming out of my office, I heard an unusual sound. I searched around to find the source. After a careful examination of the small bush that stands next to the entrance, I noticed a large robin in the thick web of its branches. She made loud chattering noises as she sat on a recently made nest.

My office building is located on a very busy street; the cars pass by in a continuous stream, producing a constant noise that made the bird's choice of sites for the upbringing of its offspring quite unexpected to me. Nevertheless, even a brief observation of the mother bird's behavior was enough to confirm that she was creating pandemonium in order to distract any outsider's attention from her little babies that lay in the nest.

The next day I waited patiently inside my office and watched the bird through the glass door. When my new neighbor finally flew away to do some errands, I came out with a ladder and climbed up to the nest. I looked inside and saw a small miracle of creation: three newly hatched nestlings were huddled closely together.

Over the next month I was able to watch how quickly the young birds developed, receiving their lessons in life not only from their mother, with whom I had first become acquainted, but from their father as well.

Nearly every day I observed how father robin and mother robin worked together in harmony, taking turns in making their constant expeditions to provide food for their children. On one balmy afternoon I was privileged to witness the first successful flight of one of the babies into the boundless blue sky.

One of the most memorable scenes I observed with the robin family was when both parents sat on the gutter of the roof above their bush loudly discussing some hot topic. I then noticed that the birds were carrying the catch of the day in their beaks—a large, fat worm—and I suddenly realized that I could discern the reason for their noisy chatter: it was a parental discussion on how to fairly divide two worms among three babies.

One warm August day the bird family was gone, leaving behind an empty nest and my unforgettable memories of their unconditional parental love. If parental love can be so unselfish in the animal kingdom, it should be so much more so among humans.

I am glad that I had the chance to document the birds' story with the many photographs that now hang on my office walls. They remind me of an episode from my own childhood. I was about six years old when, one lovely, quiet evening, my mother read me a poem by Kornei Chukovsky, one of the most popular children's authors of the Soviet Union. The poem tells the story of a horrible monster, a malicious cockroach, who threatens to take away the children from every animal family. My mother read the lines:

> And what mother in the whole wide world
> Would ever willingly give away
> Her dear little child—
> Her little bear, her little wolf, her little
> elephant. . .

At this line tears streamed from my eyes, and my mother tenderly patted my back with her warm, loving hand. No one had ever taught me, nor had I ever been told what I intuitively felt at that moment—the child's awe-inspiring realization that his mother would never give him up.

I have since found confirmation of my childhood intuition in innumerable pieces of art. In all human cultures maternal love is seen as the holiest of holies. Many works of art portray scenes where a parent—usually the mother, less frequently the father—is, due to dire circumstances, forced to abandon a child. In these scenes the event is depicted as a major heartrending tragedy of indescribable magnitude for both the parent and the child. How much this contrasts with the sometimes cold-blooded and calculating, sometimes completely mindless and irresponsible attitude that surrounds modern-day child abandonment.

Of course, all parents must, sooner or later, begin to encourage their children to leave the safe haven of the family in search of the new horizons of the wide world. Also, there are, no doubt, some situations in which a parent has no choice but to separate from a child. All too often in the cases I have observed, however, the parents who abandoned their child and ignored their natural responsibility to their own flesh and blood did so for doubtful and selfish reasons.

A HAPPY FATHER

IT REQUIRES no knowledge of the precise statistics of child abandonment to realize that far more men than women abandon their children. Due to the bond of pregnancy a mother par excellence is biologically closer to a child and her maternal instinct, to our understanding, should unconditionally guarantee that she would build an impenetrable bulwark between her child and all of life's troubles and dangers. That makes it seem much more shocking and dramatic when a mother leaves her child, and betrays this precept.

At any given moment in my pediatric practice, there are several families in which a child is being raised by a single father. As a rule, however, there is also an involved paternal grandmother who, together with her son, provides an abundance of tender love and gentle care to the baby.

One such father, Rex Hinsley, was referred to my practice by his internist, a good friend of mine.

At thirty years of age Rex was a happy man. His good-natured smile seldom left his amiable, kind face, but when he held his daughter his face shone with visible pleasure. Rex worked as a photographer for a small camera store that he owned with his cousin.

Since he had started coming to our office, he had not missed a single appointment for his child. All of these appointments for Glenna were well-baby checkups—fortunately, she was never sick. Rex would usually bring the baby by himself, but on one or two occasions his mother came along. Looking at Rex's mother, it was easy to figure out from whom he had inherited his boundless kindness. A smile similar to Rex's warmed her pleasant face.

As usual, Glenna was brought to the office on this date for a well-baby visit. Glenna at nine months of age was a beautiful darling, dressed in her colorful clothes. After she was examined and had received her necessary immunizations, the visit was practically over. Glenna was beginning to stop her whining from the pain of her shots when I noticed that Rex was consoling his daughter with some tender words.

"Take it easy, Rex," I comforted him. "The pain is already gone. In a second she will be happy again. Really, you look just like a typical overprotective mother."

By nature Mr. Hinsley was a quiet, soft-spoken man. What he could not verbalize was usually emphatically expressed in his open, animated face.

"Somebody has to do it, Doc," he said—a phrase I have heard so many times from dedicated parents. "At this moment I wish that her mother were here, but she's gone," Rex continued.

He then told me the story of his wife, who had left him and their child when the baby was about three months old. They had been married for about two years. After a small quarrel his wife, Hilda, told him that she couldn't take it any more; she quickly packed a couple of suitcases and disappeared from their apartment. Rex was sure that she would return, but the months passed, and Hilda did not come back. Rex then found out from his friends that Hilda was living with another man Rex had never heard about. He later discovered that he was not Hilda's first husband, as she had claimed, but her second husband and that their daughter was Hilda's third child. In circumstances similar to those in which she had left Rex and Glenna, she had left a son and a daughter with her first husband.

"I can hardly fathom parents who abandon their children," I said to Rex. "At least tell me what kind of person she was."

"Doc, you would never have thought that she would do such a thing. But I guess I can understand it. She has been on alcohol and drugs, especially heroin, for quite some time. That screws up your mind—no question about it."

"I can understand that she was somehow able to hide from you that she had a husband before you and that from this marriage she had two children, whom she had abandoned, but, from what I have just heard from you, it was clear to you that she was a serious drug and alcohol user. Couldn't you expect some serious complications in your marriage with these kinds of problems?"

For a short time his smile left Rex's face.

"You're 100 percent right, Doctor," he said, lowering his voice, "but you see, nobody is perfect. After I had lost my father I became involved with drugs myself. For four years I could not regain control over my destiny. I made my life and my mother's life miserable. Then I decided to quit. I got enrolled in a long-term drug rehabilitation facility. There I met Glenna's mother. I did well after rehabilitation, and I thought my wife would be rehabilitated as well. I was wrong. Whatever was helpful in it for me did not work for her."

Unexpectedly, his wonderful smile returned to his face and illuminated it.

"Doc, don't feel sorry for me. I don't regret what happened a bit. Yes, she abandoned her daughter and left me. But look what she left behind—she left behind the greatest present, the greatest miracle I could dream of—my little Glenna. I know you might think it strange, but I am grateful to her for that."

BONDING

ONE MORE child was born to this world in one of the university hospitals, where I was on staff. I was informed about it late in the evening by a nurse from the nursery. On the next day, early in the morning, I examined Baby Girl Weiss and found her healthy and charming. Buoyed with the pleasant feeling that follows an encounter with a new life, I went to the parents' room to tell them the good news.

Marian, the mother of the newborn, was thirty-six years old and her husband, Terry, was three years older. The Weiss family belonged to the white-collar middle class. Three large bouquets of flowers stood on the bedside table, and several bright-pink balloons proclaimed, "It's a Girl" as they floated against the ceiling.

Though the parents were glad to hear that their newborn child was in great shape, their reaction was somehow flat, as if they took it for granted that nothing could be wrong with their little girl.

I had never met the Weisses before; therefore, I introduced myself and told them about my office and my staff. The Weisses, who had been married about two years then told me a little about themselves. Before their marriage both of them had been divorced. The newborn was Marian's third child, but Terry's first.

I then asked Marian about her plans for the baby's feeding. She had completed her Lamaze classes and knew that breast-feeding would result in a closer bond between mother and child, so she was determined to pursue this method. Naturally I welcomed her decision and we discussed some of the issues related to it.

Our conversation was cordial, and I asked Marian about her children's reaction to the newcomer. Were they excited and impatient to see their younger sister?

"Sure, sure," answered Marian.

Marian and Terry, with their open, sincere faces and positive attitudes, presented themselves as caring people, typical of the parents I meet all the time. Maybe Marian's eye contact was not very strong, but, after all, she was probably tired and in pain from her delivery.

The Weisses had only recently bought a house in the same neighborhood where I had been practicing pediatrics for several years. Besides her newborn child, Marian had a seven-year-old son and a three-year-old daughter. I asked Marian to tell me more about her older children, about their health and personalities, and whether she and her husband planned to have me take care of their other children as well.

"Of course, Doctor, our children will use your services, but only my daughters will be your patients. Bobby, my son, lives with his father, my ex-husband," Marian answered, raising her voice a little bit as if she wanted to hear her own explanation. She smiled hesitantly, and I saw a trace of guilt in her gray eyes. To suppress "a small, little voice" inside her chest, she spoke louder and finished with enthusiasm. "When we were dividing everything during our divorce our lawyers told us that as far as children are concerned the simplest arrangement will be to divide them between my ex and me: Bobby, the oldest child went to live with my husband, and my daughter, Suzy, the younger one, went to live with me. Both my ex and I thought that this was good advice."

As I listened to Marian, I realized that she was speaking about a major decision that had been made for her family by an outsider.

I remembered an episode from my own childhood. When I was seven, I contracted measles, and though it was not a severe case of this potentially serious infection, nevertheless, the disease did completely erase my memory of a couple days of my life. When I returned to consciousness, the first thing I saw was the soft light that fell on my face from the lamp on my desk and my mother, bathed in this soft glow, as she sat next to my bed. She looked at me, and an unforgettable smile was on her face when I opened my eyes. The warmth and love I felt at that moment is one of my most precious memories.

In similar circumstances one of Marian's children was much less likely to find his mother at his bedside. How could a stranger even with the best intentions, know for certain what was better for children, and how could the parents plead advice from an outsider as a leading cause in decision which should be their sole responsibility?

Can anyone really replace a mother or a father who is still alive and well but only pops in and out to see her or his child from time to time? Though Marian did not live far from the house where she had left her son, would she be on hand when he hurt his finger or woke in the middle of the night with a nightmare?

In each life conflict, there is a winner and a loser. Adults may win or lose as a result of the drama of a divorce, but the children cannot win when one of their parents leaves their immediate environment, the family. Continuous human contact, its warmth, immediacy and availability, is replaced by less direct and tangible ways of communication.

I wondered whether, seven years earlier when Marian's son was born, she had been as concerned about bonding with him through natural childbirth methods and breast-feeding as she was today with her newborn daughter.

To understand and to feel that parent-child bond, the strongest of all human bonds, parents can follow Lamaze or other bond-forming methods, but the most important way to form a bond is simply to listen to the faithful voice of their human hearts.

LIVING EASY, LIVING FREE

I HAD known Darla Melchor from the time I was on staff at Doctors' Community Hospital. At that time she was only twenty-three years old and was working as a transcriber in the medical transcription department, where dictation is made to a hard copy. Darla was doing transcriptions for the pediatric floor. I preferred not to dictate over the phone, but directly to the tape-recorder. This made me a frequent visitor to the transcription department, where I met Darla, and gradually become well acquainted with her. Darla had a memorable personality: even when very busy, she was agreeable, attentive, and polite. When asked a question, she never pretended that she had not heard it; when she promised to do something, she did not forget about it.

Though she had no background in art or design, she had a talent for interior decoration. For Christmas and other occasions she was responsible for decorating the walls and corridors, and she always received kudos for the great job she did.

On the other hand, Darla was a little bossy and never missed a chance to demonstrate her importance to the unit. She did not take criticism well, and when something was not going her way, she would become silent and withdrawn.

Darla was tall and carried herself well. Though she could not be called beautiful, she was attractive, and her big, chocolate-brown eyes were remarkable. With the years Darla had gained weight, and this gradually caused her to lose her shapely figure. Only her face retained its slender contours.

Darla had once taken some classes in interior decoration at a local community college, and, sometimes, when she needed money, she offered her services in this field. Years before, I had invited her to wallpaper some examining rooms at my office. Though I had asked only Darla, she, to my surprise, came with her boyfriend, David. They both worked with little enthusiasm and, ignoring the presence of my staff and families of patients, periodically became embroiled in heated arguments. Eventually, I asked them to concentrate more on their work and not be so loud.

When the day was over, Darla asked for a disproportionately large payment, explaining that she had factored in the value of her boyfriend's help. I gave her no argument as I paid her in full, but I never again asked Darla to work in my office.

Some time later I saw Darla at the transcription unit, and she had a nasty black eye. She told me without hesitation when I asked what had happened that the black eye had been given to her by David, who beat her up when they "got into a fight." A month later Darla had another black eye—the cause was the same as before. Periodically Darla made peace with her assaulter: apparently, in spite of the violence, it was important to Darla to keep her steady boyfriend.

Darla and I had known each other for more than four years when she decided to leave the transcription unit; she wanted something more challenging than just typing reports. At her request, she was transferred to work as a clerk in the emergency room.

The new job meant we no longer had occasion to meet as frequently as we had before, but whenever I did see Darla, she was still as happy and full of energy as ever.

One fine spring day, while going to a patient's room, I entered the hospital elevator where, among the other passengers, I noticed Darla. To my big surprise her belly was noticeably enlarged, and I realized that she was pregnant. We left the elevator, and I congratulated her on the expected birth of her child. She accepted my best wishes with a generous, amiable smile. It was lunchtime, and we decided to have lunch in the cafeteria and catch up on one another.

Over lunch Darla told me that she still could not reconcile with David, the father of her child, because he "was not serious enough." I did not even dare to mention the word "marriage" in our conversation: Darla was happy that at the very least she had not had a fight with David for the preceding four months.

Darla was not daunted by the idea of becoming a single mother; when I asked her about the future, she did not want to go into that prosaic matter and switched the conversation to another topic.

Darla was expecting her baby in a couple of weeks; she solemnly promised to let me know when the baby was born.

Two weeks later, while I was on my morning rounds in the newborn nursery at the University of Illinois Hospital, I noticed an attractive, plump baby girl who lay in her crib diligently working on a pacifier. This cute baby's last name was Melchor.

I needed no explanation and rushed to Darla's room to share in her joy at the birth of her wonderful daughter. Darla looked content and sweet as always. She answered my excited remarks with a weak and polite smile. Surprised at the lack of enthusiasm on her part, I asked her how she was feeling. Darla gave me the usual answer that is given by most women after a delivery: she was still sore, but other than that she was fine.

I complimented her on her daughter's appearance and asked what she was planning to name the baby. Darla's answer was no less surprising to me than my discovery two weeks earlier that she was pregnant. In a very matter-of-fact way, she told me that the baby's name was not on her agenda as she was not going to be her baby for very much longer.

With an air of importance, she spoke with me as if I were a person who, in these modern times of individual freedom, could share her outlook on life and easily appreciate her mature decision, which she took for granted I would approve. "Besides," she concluded, trying to demonstrate her practical wisdom, "besides, I am not ready for a baby."

"What do you mean, 'I am not ready for a baby'?" I asked Darla, my former friend. "You have a baby!"

"My relationship with David is still unsettled." Darla started to enumerate her reasons for giving up her newborn baby. "I need to save some money to buy a house, as I planned. Besides, I'm not done with college yet: I've got to get my interior design diploma."

In her twenty-seventh year of life Darla Melchor was not yet ready to become a mother to her newborn daughter. She was giving the child away to a childless couple with whom she had recently become acquainted. Sadness, sorrow, or pain? None of it was in Darla's voice. Instead, she demonstrated something familiar to me from other, similar cases—a subdued pride for having made such good accommodations for her baby. As fantastic as it may sound, it appeared that Darla saw the abandonment of her child as the performance of a positive social function: as a conscientious, caring citizen, she was generously providing a child to an infertile couple.

After this meeting at the hospital, I tried to make my subsequent encounters with Darla as brief as possible. I don't know whether she realized the reason for my lack of desire to maintain a conversation with her. Our talks now consisted of a few polite, empty phrases.

Darla called my office about two years after our meeting in her hospital room. Again she surprised me—this time by telling me that she had been fired from her job at the hospital. Darla was her usual candid self. The reason for her dismissal was her late arrival for work. I did not ask her the reason for her tardiness, but she volunteered it anyway.

"You know," she told me, "I live far from the hospital."

Darla was silent when, unable to resist, I softly suggested to her that she could rent an apartment around the hospital in order to be on time for work. The other logical suggestion—that she could wake up earlier if she really wanted to be on time—I kept to myself, as I did not want to make her too uncomfortable.

Darla then told me the reason for her call. She was in trouble. The hospital was not willing to gloss over the reason for her dismissal, and this considerably reduced her chances for finding a new job. In addition to letting me know that she was using me as a reference, Darla was also asking me "to bend the truth a little" and help her fudge her employment history of the last ten years.

I told Darla that I would be happy to confirm the fact that I knew her but that I could not permit her to state that she had been working in my office for the last decade.

When Darla asked why I refused, I gave her an excuse that should have been familiar to her; two years earlier, when she was abandoning her baby, she had told me that she was not ready for her child; now I told her that, though I was sorry, I was not ready to do what she was asking of me—I was not ready for a lie.

Whether she recognized these words as her own I can't say, but it was obvious that she was ready for my refusal and had only been hoping that I would allow her deception.

"Anyway," she said in conclusion, "I gave you as a reference."

I abstained from further comment, though Darla had not asked for my permission to use my name as a reference and had told me of it as a fait accompli.

She never called me again.

PERFECT ABANDONMENT, OR, UTERUS FOR HIRE

FAITH MOBERLEY, a single mother in her early twenties, was using the services of our pediatric office not only for her six-year-old daughter, Jill, but for herself as well. She had been sixteen and had no parental support when Jill was born at Doctors' Community Hospital.

Two weeks later she brought her to my office for a well-baby checkup. Since then Jill and, later, Faith, had become regular patients in our practice. Faith, who was still in the age range for pediatric practice, was treated by us after her numerous requests for help with her frequent bronchitis and ear infections. Her heavy smoking contributed to her illnesses.

I had never met Jill's father. To the best of my knowledge, he abandoned Faith even before she told him that she was pregnant with Jill. Faith was a longtime public aid recipient.

Jill had been a very big girl since her birth. She was developing well, but, perhaps because of her mother's irregular lifestyle, she got a lot of colds and upper-respiratory tract infections. At the age of four she developed bronchial asthma, fortunately, of a mild kind.

To her mother's credit, she never missed a single appointment for her daughter and was careful to give her prescribed medicines.

Faith frequently took Jill to the emergency room of the local hospital. From the emergency room's slips, I knew that she usually showed up there around 3 o'clock in the morning—the time when she was returning home from her evening activities. My questions as to what she was doing at such a late hour were met with silence. I had my own theories about her pastimes, but I never had enough evidence to suspect her of something truly reprehensible.

It was strange that even though Faith took good care of her body, there were, more frequently than not, dark stripes that looked like dirt under her poorly manicured fingernails.

In addition to public aid benefits, Faith received food stamps, which she put to good use—gradually, with each passing year, her formerly lean body became more and more plump, though she was never really obese.

Faith had a sexual appeal of an animal variety, which she did not lose even after the features of her large face, which were never too fine, became rather coarse, and her blue, bovine eyes gradually lost their youthful brilliance.

Faith hardly ever maintained eye contact for more than one or two seconds; our conversations usually consisted of my doing a monologue. Faith, when questioned, would break her silence with an answer that rarely consisted of more than four or five words. She was also poor at expressing her feelings—I had never seen any evidence of either delight or displeasure on her emotionless face.

Even though Faith hid behind a wall of seeming indifference, I respected her for the care and attention she gave to her daughter.

One day, however, Faith broke her silence. She had apparently overheard my conversation with a medical assistant as we talked about Mrs. Kay's adopted baby. Mr. and Mrs. Kay had waited for several years to get this adorable child.

When the medical assistant left the room, Faith looked at me with her prominent eyes and asked if she could talk to me about something. I expressed my interest and invited her to sit down.

"Doc," she said, "can I be honest with you?"

I assured Faith of the confidentiality of our talk.

"Doc," Faith continued in the hoarse voice of a heavy smoker, "you know a lot of people who might want to have babies. If there was a woman who could not, you know, get pregnant, then I might be for hire to get the baby for that couple. Don't worry about money—I wouldn't ask for much."

Faith was not upset when I expressed my disinterest in her offer; the permanent emotionless expression returned to her face.

A year later Faith stopped coming to the office without notice or any request for the transfer of Jill's medical record.

Do I condemn Faith for offering her body for insemination by some unknown man and then using her uterus as an incubator for the growth and development of a fetus that she would eventually relinquish to some infertile couple?

No, I cannot condemn her. She was simply following the trends of the contemporary society in which she lives. The predictions given in Aldous Huxley's *Brave New World* have not yet, fortunately for humankind, been realized; however, the exotic aspects of artificial insemination are dangerously meddling with fundamental issues of the origin of human life—the greatest of miracles, a miracle we share in but did not create. The consequences of such meddling with this, hidden behind seven seals, sacrament, are yet unknown.

Faith's offer reflects the current brave new world's cavalier attitude to the holiness and mystery of life. I am sure that she saw no element of child abandonment in her offer; she was merely proposing to deliver some merchandise, which happened to be a human being. Faith's only worry was to hide her intentions of directly charging money for her services from the authorities, as this is illegal.

DOUBLE STANDARDS

WHILE LOOKING at the open, innocent face and cordial appearance of Sue Rucker at the end of a visit to my office, I recalled a line from the Roman writer of fables, Phædrus, "Things are not always what they seem." Sue and her then one-year-old daughter were patients in my office on the near-West side of Chicago where I worked prior to my present location. Initially, my pediatric clientele numbered too few to provide a living, so I took care of adults as well. Sue Rucker was the mother of the first newborn in this practice. She suffered from respiratory allergies, and, between visits for her own problems and well-visits for her newborn baby, I saw her a lot.

One day, to my surprise, I found Sue in the exam room with two children whom I had never met before: eleven-year-old Clementina and seven-year-old Lindsey, as I learned from the medical charts. They had different last names from that of Sue and her young child, my regular patients.

I am not sure if Sue noticed me when I entered the room, but both children continued with their own activities and totally ignored my presence. They breezed from one corner of the room to the other, sometimes talking to each other, sometimes jumping up, sometimes laughing loudly. I soon noticed that they paid little attention to Sue as she sat and quietly observed them. She seemed to be neither involved with, nor affected, by the chaotic commotion the youngsters produced.

Sue Rucker looked at least five years younger than her thirty years. The soft, maternal smile that she had worn on her previous visits was present today as well. Expressing my surprise at seeing these children, whom I had never seen with her before, I asked her who they were.

"These are my children, Doctor. They came for an exam and just to get acquainted with you. Can you check them over?" she answered quickly. From her tone I understood that she did not want to be questioned further.

Soon the exam was over. After handing the forms to each of Sue's children—who, in response to my delicate requests, behaved in a much more appropriate manner—I asked them to leave the room. In their absence, I asked Sue why I had never met her older children before, even though she had been coming into my office for a long time.

"You shouldn't be surprised, Doctor," she answered earnestly and sincerely. "This is the first time in the last four years that I've seen them myself. I just picked them up from their father and brought them over to you for a checkup."

She became silent but, probably realizing that she needed to give me more of an explanation, continued.

"The child you usually see is from my second marriage. My first marriage was a disaster. When we were going through our divorce, we decided that the children would stay with their father and I would move out. Actually, I intended to leave them with him for only a couple of months, but then my ex sued me for custody and, as a result, the children went to him."

I told Sue that, to the best of my knowledge in cases involving custody rights, the court usually gives priority to the mother rather than the father. How was it that for such a reliable person and law-abiding citizen as Sue, the court came to this rather unusual decision?

"First of all," Sue answered trustingly, "he was making a lot more money than me; second, he had a mother who was helping him to take care of the kids; and, besides, he had a two-bedroom apartment and I had only one bedroom.

"I thought it over and moved to an apartment several blocks away from my husband's house. In order not to confuse or upset the children, we decided that I should not contact them. Then my ex-husband and I thought that would be better for them."

I nodded, letting Sue know that I had heard all that she said, and then asked her why she had changed her mind and met her children today.

Sue gave a sigh of relief—she was over the unpleasant part of the conversation; now it was not about her and her decisions, but about her ex-husband.

"Their father was always on drugs, which was one of the reasons for our divorce," she told me confidingly, "but now it has gotten out of hand. The man has lost control of himself—he uses alcohol and drugs all the time.

"He was never very gentle with the children, but recently he started beating them, sometimes even with a belt, and as often as every other day. The neighbors complained, and the Department of Children and Family Services contacted me. I decided to take them to my house." Sue concluded without demonstrating any overwhelming emotions.

At this moment Clementina and Lindsey threw open the door and loudly asked how much longer they were going to have to wait. Sue stood up to leave.

While we were parting, I asked Sue about her present husband's reaction to her decision.

"He is more than happy that we can help them. He simply does not believe that what my ex-husband was doing to them was possible," she concluded, this time demonstrating a moderate degree of righteous indignation about her ex-husband's actions.

She left the room with her children, and I thought about how she would react if it were not she, but, instead, her ex-husband who had not seen his own children for even a visit in four long years, who had not sent a note or even made a phone call to them, though he had been living in the same suburb all these years.

Judge not, that ye be not judged.

ANOTHER CAMILLE

ALMOST TWENTY years ago, I was doing my pediatric residency at a large medical center in Chicago. Early one morning, when I was on rotating shifts in the newborn nursery, baby girl Heisler was born to her eighteen-year-old mother, Camille. Camille had been having frequent uterine contractions in the middle of the night, when her boyfriend brought her to the emergency room. She was taken to labor and delivery almost immediately, and two hours later gave birth to a healthy, outstandingly pretty child whom she refused to touch, to see, or even to hear about.

Camille belonged to a group of mothers who abdicate their parental responsibilities and rights immediately after their child's birth. This group consists of people with different characters and different social positions; many are young and poor.

Life is hard; without a doubt, some of the mothers who abandon their children are in tremendously difficult circumstances. Over the years, however, I have observed another group, who abandon their newborn babies on a regular basis every two to three years and simply want to get rid of the child.

Camille belonged to the latter category. Though she had not made a single prenatal visit with a physician, she had, nevertheless, visited a private adoption agency three days before her delivery and made all of the necessary arrangements for the adoption to take place. She casually informed the medical personnel of this before she was taken to labor and delivery.

In her eighteenth year, Camille looked like a beautiful angel— she was delicate, fragile looking, and, yes, she was bashful. Only the numerous multicolored tattoos on her body and her nicotine-stained fingers betrayed her irregular lifestyle. The records showed that her two previous pregnancies had ended with abortions.

Camille had stated on several occasions that she wanted to be discharged from the hospital as soon as possible. In the early morning of the day after her delivery, Dr. Baldwin, who had delivered Camille's baby, entered her room, checked her over, and then told her that she could go home immediately.

"Thank you, Doc," Camille said as she flashed him an innocent smile.

"Do you have any questions?" Dr. Baldwin inquired.

"Only one, Doc," replied Camille softly. "When can I resume having sex?"

Usually adopted children disappear from the pediatrician's life forever as soon as they are discharged from the hospital to their adoptive parents. With Camille's baby, however, this was not the case.

Two weeks later, I entered an exam room at the newborn clinic, and saw a baby in the company of her two happy parents, who were in their early forties.

Without giving me a chance to speak, the father, a tall, robust man, asked me with a shining smile, "Doctor, do you recognize this girl?"

I looked at the baby and immediately recognized Camille's outstandingly pretty daughter. Stunned, as I had never expected to see this child again, I looked on, unable to say a word.

"Doctor, we had tried to adopt a baby for the last five years. I hope you have no doubts that this child is now in good hands."

"What did you name your baby?" I asked the happy father.

"We called her Camille, Doctor. But she is going to be a different Camille."

"I don't doubt it," I answered carefully, trying to control my emotions—little Camille was in good hands.

We live in a small world. Recently, young parents came with their two-month-old daughter for the first visit to my office. It is routine to ask the family who referred them. "Oh, yes," answered the mother, a lovely young woman, giving me a shining smile. "My parents recognized your name in the insurance book. They recently moved to Florida."

"My name is Camille," she continued after a short pause. "You took care of me in the pediatric clinic of Doctors' Hospital."

"Camille," I repeated mechanically. "It's such a long time since I was a pediatric resident there. Can you give some clue?"

"You used to call me 'Another Camille' when I was a baby, my mother said..." began my old-time patient.

She did not need to continue. Of course I remembered the little Camille, who, thanks to her adaptive parents, was given a chance for a normal, clean, good life. Her parents kept their promise.

SOCIAL RESPONSIBILITY

THOUGH I had never met Michelle Anderson before this visit, I had heard more than enough about her from her father, who was a good friend of mine. Michelle, at her young age, had two children, one of whom was three, and the other, five. They had both been born out of wedlock and were by different fathers.

Michelle's father, Walter, owned a small grocery store. He and I played racquetball twice a week at the local health club. Walter and his wife, Sylvia, a charming and energetic woman, had two daughters— Michelle and Madeline, who were twenty-one and nineteen years old, respectively. Unlike Michelle, Madeline had never presented any problems for her parents—she was a warm and responsible person who was now studying at a local college.

If Madeline was a great help to her parents, Michelle had been a constant worry to them since the time she was twelve. First it was her academic achievements, or lack thereof; later it was her behavior. At the age of sixteen Michelle left her family; Walter or Sylvia would see her from time to time, usually unexpectedly, in many different places—on the street, at the mall, or when she would come back home for a short period of time.

The major problems with Michelle began after she gave birth to her children, Nathaniel and Karen. Neither Walter nor Sylvia could ignore what was happening with their grandchildren. Despite their efforts Michelle was a very irresponsible mother who continued to spend her time "partying" with her numerous acquaintances. After several instances in which she had abandoned her children—either by leaving them for several days with different friends or leaving them alone at home—and after giving solid proof that she was a serious drug addict, a judge granted Walter and Sylvia's request for custody of Nathaniel when he was six months old and then, two years later, of Karen when she was ten months old.

Neither Walter nor Sylvia were really looking for another chance to return to their younger years and raise small children. But they were normal people—instead of stones in their chest they had the hearts of a human being and responded to the suffering of those around them, especially their own flesh and blood—and they simply could not stand by and allow their grandchildren to suffer from a poor environment and their mother's neglect.

Since Nathaniel had come to live with Walter and Sylvia, even before he was officially adopted by them, he had become a regular patient in my office. Later and in similar circumstances, Karen joined her older brother at the Anderson house and at my pediatric practice.

Walter had come to my office for a visit with both of his grandchildren about three weeks before his daughter appeared for her first and, thus far, only visit to my office. Walter had never lost hope that one fine day his daughter was going to become a responsible person. Thus, though he and Sylvia had full custody of both children, not only was Michelle allowed, but she was, in fact, welcomed to visit her children and to take them with her whenever she wanted. She exercised this opportunity only minimally, however, and even then she spent time only with her younger child, Karen. She would take Karen to her house once in a while for a couple of days but practically ignored the existence of her older son.

During this last visit Walter, by nature a talkative and friendly person, was unusually silent. I could remember him being so silent only when he was in the process of adopting his grandchildren. We were in close terms, so at the end of the visit I asked him the reason for his unhappiness.

"It's Michelle, Vladimir," Walter answered in an irritated manner. "It's her and her irresponsibility. I just found out that she is pregnant again, this time again by another boyfriend. She expects to have the baby in three or four months.

"I told her," he was whispering emphatically to me as he did not want Nathaniel and Karen to hear him, "that this time we will not take care of the child. No way! She practically abandoned these children when they lived with her. She can't go a day without cocaine, and then she expects Sylvia and me to clean up after her messes.

Walter raised his voice, "No, way! I will let *her* deal with her own child; Sylvia and I are not going to step in this time. No way! I told her that this child is her responsibility, not ours. Enough is enough."

There was nothing new in Walter's emotional outburst: he had reacted the same way before he adopted the first two children. I could bet all my money that once he and Sylvia got acquainted with their new grandchild, their hearts would melt with a warm wave of love, and they would inevitably begin caring for the new baby as well. Before that, Michelle would disappear—for a party where she would use drugs or for some short-lived passion—sometimes for a day, sometimes for a week, and she would leave the new baby with some neighbors or a girlfriend. The new child will eventually join his two siblings at his grandparents' house. The Andersons will forget about their resolution to let Michelle pay the consequences of her lack of responsibility. They would not allow their grandchild to become a ward of the state and enter the foster child care system.

Two weeks later I met Walter at the health club. To my questions about Michelle, he told me that he and Sylvia thought that Michelle had taken a step in the right direction: she had been clean and sober for the last week. She had also taken Karen to live with her and was, so far, taking good care of her.

Three days later Michelle called my office to arrange an appointment for Karen.

That evening Michelle and Karen were waiting for me in one of the exam rooms. We exchanged greetings as if we were old acquaintances. Though she knew that I was well informed about her behavior, there was no hint of guilt or shame in her manner; if she had these feelings, they were hidden very deeply in her subconscious, which she had been anesthetizing with alcohol and drugs.

Though she was a chronic substance abuser, this was hardly noticeable on her face—its destructive force had not yet started to leave its mark on her. Moreover, despite her chosen way of life, the overpowering force of youth still preserved Michelle's natural attractiveness and spontaneity.

The visit did not present any surprises. If I did not know about Michelle's history of child abandonment I would never have suspected anything unusual in her relations with Karen, who was peacefully playing with the toys that lay in front of her on the floor.

Karen was only slightly sick. I wrote a prescription for a decongestant, and Michelle came up to the desk to pick it up from me. The proportions of her young body and the size of her stomach could easily be considered normal, but Walter could not be wrong.

Michelle knew all too well that I was a part of the network of enablers who were dealing with the results of her conduct. This gave me the right to ask her straight out if she was pregnant.

My question did not catch Michelle off guard. She looked at me as if she had something very important to say.

"Well, I have good news and bad news. Where do you want me to start?" she said with a winsome smile.

"Start with the bad," I suggested.

"The bad news is that, yes, I am pregnant . . . But I have good news as well." Michelle paused solemnly, as if preparing me for words of comfort and hope.

"The good news is that my gynecologist (she pronounced it gahnah-cah-logist) told me that I have something wrong with my ovaries. Which means . . ."

Another, longer pause followed. "Which means," Michelle concluded victoriously, "that in the future I *might* not be able to have more children!"

"Amen," came out of my mouth against my will. "Tell it to your parents. They might rejoice in your sense of social responsibility."

Michelle answered me with a wry smile but said nothing.

ONLY SIX HOURS APART

CONNIE HOBART, a respiratory therapist, was a good friend of mine. We were brought together during a cold, long, difficult January night on the pediatric floor of Doctors' Community Hospital, when we took care of a five-year-old child severely sick with bronchial asthma. By morning, not only had our patient improved, but also we had learned that we could really rely on each other.

Connie was happily married. The Hobart family lived in a northern suburb of Chicago. I did not realize that Connie had an eighteen-year-old daughter until she called my office and told me that her daughter, Lena, expected to have a baby in about a month. Connie wanted me to be her future grandchild's pediatrician, but did not say much about her daughter. All I knew was that Lena planned to continue living with her parents and that constant conflicts had caused her to break up with her boyfriend, the father of her child.

About a month later, Lena and her mother came in with the newborn child, who had been born in a community hospital where I was not on staff. Lena was very nice looking, intelligent, and cordial. She was bustling around her new daughter, Violet, as if she were an experienced mother. Connie was trying to assist the young mother by handing her a diaper, clothes, creams, and wipes.

Lena was happy to talk with me about her adjustment to motherhood. She was sincerely hoping to be both a good student and a good mother. After Violet's birth Lena stopped attending the school for pregnant teens and immediately returned to her own school, where the academic requirements were much higher. She was determined to remain on the honor roll, as she had been since the first grade. It was easy for me to believe her; she looked like a future professional: a lawyer, a doctor, or, perhaps, a college professor.

Lena's school and church began using her as a role model. Soon the largest Chicago newspapers had published the story of the teen mother who was unwilling to give up and was determined to keep striving for her future career. Lena appeared not only on Chicago television programs but also on national networks as well.

She was still bringing her daughter to my office on a regular basis. I found that her celebrity status had not changed her at all—she remained as pleasant and modest as ever. I saw Lena's name in the different newspaper and magazine articles, and soon began to notice a common denominator in the coverage dedicated to her: they all discussed Lena's career plans and her academic success, but none of them dealt with Lena's role as the mother of a child.

Lena lives in an industrial society whose priority is to create and produce a skilled workforce. Seeing human beings and their families in a spiritual light is above and beyond the primary interest of this society. I was trying to stay within the circle of Lena's admirers, and did my best to repress these killjoy thoughts, which made me feel vaguely guilty about my poorly confirmed misgivings.

The last time I saw Lena in my office was when she came in for an appointment for her daughter, who was at that time six months old. Violet was very advanced for her age; she was well developed both physically and psychologically. Lena looked very nice and was smartly dressed. She shone with the exuberance of youth.

After Violet had been examined, Lena and I began to chat. Lena, with modest pride, told me that she had graduated from high school cum laude. I congratulated her and asked her about her plans.

"I was accepted by several universities, but I chose the University of Cincinnati," Lena told me happily. "I am going to study international trade there," she finished, while gathering the baby's things together and putting them into the diaper bag.

I congratulated Lena again and, holding Violet's little hand in mine, asked, "What is going to happen to this little one? Where are you going to live with her? How are you going to make it without your parents' help?"

Lena answered me with a smile—she was happy to let me know that she had thought it all through.

"No. Violet is going to stay with my parents. They are more than happy to take care of her. Meanwhile, I will have enough time to achieve my goals. I'll still come home to see Violet on the weekends and holidays."

The words came out of my mouth before I had a chance to think about them. "Well, you won't always be able to come home: you will have a lot of tests, exams, homework; your life will be busy. Violet will miss you a lot these next few years."

"She won't," Lena replied sincerely and without offense. "I have several friends from my town who will study with me. We are planning to come home whenever we can. After all, I am only six hours away from my daughter."

"So what?" some readers would say. After all, Lena was leaving her daughter, not with strangers, but with the infant's loving grandparents. Many mothers (and fathers) leave their children with relatives. Do I want to see Lena sitting at home with her daughter, raising her and be dependent on welfare?

Of course, I am glad that Lena is looking out for her future, but doesn't her daughter's existence place on Lena, as a mother, the responsibility for some direct—and not by correspondence—upbringing, support, and day-to-day emotional nourishment of her daughter?

If not, then what are parents for? To create children and then to place them in reliable hands? In that case, parents are nothing more than baby-making machines. It is a question of priorities: what is more important for Lena: to become a professional in the shortest possible time or to be a mother to her child?

We are not in a time of war or calamity in which people are forced to make these kinds of terrible choices. There are plenty of good universities in Chicago where Lena could study the same subjects as she could hundreds of miles from her home. Couldn't she live at home with her daughter and study at a university at the same time? Nevertheless, even such a fine sensitive person as she chose to go away and leave her daughter for four, five, or more years.

If even such a positive and exemplary person as Lena did not hesitate to leave her child behind, and if our society fully approves of this decision, then our priorities have drastically changed: the most important thing for people has become the pursuit of their careers, and the family has become a secondary occupation, a hostage to the goals and purposes of our industrial society.

The main losers are our children, whose trust is being fundamentally betrayed. If they are no longer the first priority for their own parents, how much less a priority are they for the rest of the society?

9

CHILDREN BEGETTING CHILDREN

Only in the last two centuries has the age at which women are expected to have children become so advanced in the Western world. These norms run against the general history of humans. Even now in some areas of the world procreation begins when the individuals are biologically capable of such functions. Therefore, there is nothing unnatural about a female and male of adolescent age choosing to have babies. Many happy children have been born to such families.

A serious problem that I frequently see is not the young age of the parents but the absence of any husband-wife relationship—this relationship creates the basis of the family in our society and is the unit in which children can themselves develop into future mothers and fathers. Many of the families headed by teen parents are also characterized by the sad lack of commitment to the family on the part of the father and by the unpreparedness on the part of the teenage mother for the important role of teaching societal values and cultural traditions to her children.

Many American children are born every year to teenage mothers, and the majority of these mothers are warm, caring human beings. For many, especially those sixteen years of age and older, the pregnancy was not unwanted or a surprise. These mothers love their children just as much as older mothers do, but they sometimes cannot compensate for their immaturity. Thus, children are begetting children.

The children born to these teenage mothers are usually raised by grandmothers who are frequently not very old themselves. The teen-age mothers who are more mature and independent usually raise their offspring themselves; nevertheless, these teen mothers often still live with their parents, although sometimes the baby's father may visit or even live with the girl's family. Availability of welfare benefits for teenage mothers, paradoxically, has resulted in a dearth of families through all social groups and helped to dissolve the institution of marriage among these families. In the past a woman and a man who decided to have a family were helped along by their extended families but were expected to rely on their own abilities to provide for themselves and for their child. As long as they claimed to be mature enough to have children, they were considered mature enough to earn their own money. In our times such a requirement might sound like blasphemy. Meanwhile, countless children of both sexes are growing up surrounded for their entire childhood only by women; men are guests in their world.

All children have the right to be well fed and dressed. It is absurd to deprive a child who is growing up with a teenage mother of financial assistance and medical help. Should the welfare system, instead, promote and reward the young family only when a father is around? Should society insist that marriage is desirable as long as help from society is being asked for? These are hard questions.

Several years ago a school principal with progressive ideas established a system of financial rewards for teenage girls, who had also been educated on how to prevent themselves from becoming pregnant. As long as the girls did not have babies, they were given a monthly allowance of five dollars. This program was begun only after the principal had proved, with figures, to the satisfaction of the progressive school board that it was more economical to pay the girls the money than to lose students because of pregnancy. The program was successful for the first nine months—the gestational period. The principal was a good mathematician but a poor psychologist—he did not realize that sexual behavior is the human activity that is least controllable by outside influences, and control over it cannot be bought for five dollars a month.

I hope that one of these days a solution to the problem of teen pregnancy will be found; meanwhile, it's up to the teenage children to bring up their new babies in this world—the teenagers, not society, are in control.

I know and respect many teenage mothers who take good care of their children. Sadly enough, I hardly know any teenage men who are able to live up to the challenge of being fathers to their own children. Initially, they sometimes come in with their girlfriends, but, gradually, they come less and less often and then not at all. As these fathers make themselves less and less available, grandmothers and, sometimes, grandfathers on the maternal side, who initially did their best to separate themselves from their daughter's affairs, gradually become more and more involved with the baby. They cannot help it—by this time they have usually fallen in love with their grandchild.

It would be an oversimplification to link the problem of teenage pregnancy in our country to the availability of welfare assistance; nevertheless, for the average girl older than, say, twelve or thirteen years of age, side by side with such factors as achieving status within the community, trying to add some meaning to life, and escaping from boredom, the accessibility of financial support is an additional factor in her passive decision to become a mother.

SIXTEEN PLUS TWELVE

I FEEL that I was fortunate to grow up in a nuclear family. As I have already expressed, for me the family represents the primary institution of the human race where children not only grow up and mature psychologically to become distinct personalities but also feel truly needed and protected.

It has always been my belief that the family fulfills a great psychological, emotional, and existential need in human beings. Like Antaeus, the figure from the Greek myth who renewed his strength whenever he touched his mother, the earth, a human being who is lucky enough to be born into a loving family derives from this source the strength and resilience needed to withstand the challenges of life.

After the so-called sexual revolution of the sixties and seventies, the types of families I see in my practice are very different from those of my childhood. My first encounter with the problems created by the sexual revolution was in the Soviet Union. The October revolution of 1917 introduced radical reforms to all aspects of society, including the institution of the family. As a pediatrician there, I saw the steady deterioration of the conventional, nuclear family—an irreplaceable unit of any civilized society.

I emigrated to the West in 1974, when the sexual revolution here was at its peak. Since resuming pediatric practice in the United States in 1978, I have observed daily the unrelenting erosion and decay of the institution of the American family—at least in the area where I have practiced for the last fifteen years. This might, in part, be due to demographics, but, while only seven or eight years ago I would have been surprised to see a child in my practice born to an unmarried couple, today there is nothing unusual about it.

When I enter an examining room, the patient has usually been prepared for the exam by a medical assistant. One day I was less busy than usual, and I sat in the examining room and scribbled in my notebook as I waited for the next patient. The door flew open, and a young man dressed in a bright orange shirt with a garish design on it burst into the room. His healthy face was full of energy, and he laughed loudly. His hair was done in the latest fashion in a porcupine-like manner, and a thick, golden earring dangled from his ear. I noticed a bright lipstick imprint on his childlike, rosy cheek.

Shortly after this, I heard laughter outside, and then the imprinter of the lipstick kiss ran like a gazelle into the examining room. Looking carefully at her, I recognized the kisser as my patient, Brandy Brogan. Her parents had begun bringing their children to my office six years earlier. All four of them always came to the office together regardless of who was sick.

I remembered Brandy's face because a bout with chickenpox a couple of years before had left two deep and noticeable scars on her forehead. I had never heard her speak much and never foresaw that she would behave so eccentrically in a medical office.

Brandy had a slim, pleasing figure, and on this sunny spring day, she had a shining, happy look, about her that I had never seen before. Though she retained her teenage look there was also something in her appearance of a woman who had accomplished the dream of her life.

Behaving as if I were not around, she immediately began to exchange giggles and sly, sexual looks with her boyfriend, Willard Brodack. Brandy's appearance brimmed not only with her enjoyment of life but also with pride in her own budding sexuality. A token of this personal development stood in beauty on her boyfriend's cheek. For his part, Willard visibly took pleasure in observing his accomplishment in the masculine sphere—Brandy's abdomen was substantially larger than would be expected for her tender age and graceful teenage stature. With Willard's help Brandy was five months pregnant.

Brandy's preferred provider organization required the primary physician to obtain approval number in order for a patient to be seen by a specialist. While Brandy and her boyfriend, both sixteen years of age, were enjoying themselves in my pediatric office, I was being transferred from one friendly phone message to another, with classical music on the background, each minute getting closer to the desired approval number for Brandy's request for a consultation with an obstetrician and pregnancy-related tests. So as not to ignore my visitors, I chatted with them a little.

I began by asking Willard whether he and Brandy were married— a question which I have recently become hesitant to ask, so obvious is the answer. I received a response in the negative, accompanied by some unexpected embarrassment on his part.

"You are going to get married soon, aren't you?" I continued. Willard laughed nervously, paused for a minute, and then looked at Brandy. The two of them began a series of playful silent messages back and forth. Finally, he responded, "Yeah, later we will, kind of," a phrase, that produced joyful laughter from both of them.

This answer was better than no answer at all; I indicated my satisfaction with it and asked Willard whether he had a job.

Willard forgot the presence of his sexual partner for a moment and spoke to me as if he were an adult. He pointed his finger at Brandy's expanding abdomen and said, "I don't work now, but I *got* to work." He did not know where he was going to work or what he was going to do, but he told me he was determined to work.

Brandy was not interested in this conversation; she was chewing gum and looking at the ceiling. I did not want to appear to ignore her, so I asked her who was going to help her when the baby was born.

This question caught Brandy off guard; she was not ready for such prosaic and boring issues. After a pause she answered me with the question, "What do you mean?" I explained my meaning and she exclaimed, "Oh, my ma and pa."

I turned to Willard and asked, "What about you, young man, are you going to help raise your future child as well?"

As if it went without saying, he exclaimed with bravado, "Sure, Doc. We're a family now!"

Ashamed of my insensitivity, I returned to my paperwork, and they immediately resumed their flirting. Their constant exchanges of sounds, smiles, and gestures reminded me so much of the communication of young children that it took a special effort for me to remember that these children were, in four months' time, going to become the parents of a real human being.

In this age of space exploration and amazing scientific discoveries, teenage parents like Brandy and Willard present a formidable task for social engineering. While the experts on both the political Left and Right are trying to solve this embarrassing, disastrously costly, and destructive problem at the national level, this young couple perceived the situation they found themselves in as an adult version of the child's game of playing house. The final responsibility for the "mess" would be handled not by them, but by their own parents, or by the authorities of "the nursery" in which they live, that is, by the community.

Brandy was not worried about the future of her child or herself. She belonged to the sizable group of teenagers who are becoming parents. From girlfriends who had been in similar situations, Brandy already had a good idea of what her future would be like. This future had already begun: her parents had told her that they would help to raise the baby; she was already attending a special school for pregnant teenagers and young mothers.

Once a month, she would begin receiving a check from the state of Illinois for the child's financial support and free health insurance. In addition, she would receive food stamps and free baby formula. Who can question the security that such help provides? None of us want to see Brandy's child, a full-fledged American citizen, living a life of poverty and misery.

While society had given adequate thought to the needs of Brandy's child, Brandy's consciousness as a citizen of this society approached the zero mark. Nothing can stop her from becoming pregnant in another two or three years and from repeating this pattern on a regular basis.

I remember reading some research that had reviewed numerous other research studies done on different attempts to control the rate of teenage pregnancy. After many ambitious schemes were implemented in these different research studies, in which teenagers were given sex education and behavior modification, this research discovered that the pregnancy rate in a large group of teenagers studied actually went up instead of decreasing as had been expected. Probably it is sometimes better to speak little than to speak too much.

Nobody argues that sex education is of value, but what in particular should children be taught? Can sex education be provided without teaching moral values as well? If sex education is provided on a large scale in a school, but the school is unwilling to discuss the moral values of our society—that is, the school is "embarrassed" to educate Brandy about moral issues and fears being accused of imposing a value system on her—how can this work? Could educating Brandy on one-thousand-and-one methods of birth control ever be effective if Brandy herself is not sure whether she wants to avoid getting pregnant in the first place?

A month passed after this visit. While working in one of the examining rooms adjacent to the waiting room, I heard loud noises. I looked into the waiting room and saw the Brogan family. Brandy, her mother, Matilda, and the three other Brogan children were involved in a hot argument.

Later I examined Brandy's younger brother Adam and then Brandy herself. Brandy's abdomen had grown noticeably, and her movements were not as quick and agile as they had been only a few weeks before. She continued to act as if she were proud of her accomplishment.

"Where is Willard?" I asked.

"He is in the waiting room. Lately he does not feel very comfortable sitting with children," Brandy said. She paused and then addressed her mother with a conspiratorial smile. "He's not going to get away from us that easy, right, Mom?" Both mother and daughter chuckled at this remark.

I expressed my interest in the family situation, and Brandy told me in a low voice that Willard, who for a short time had lived with her at her parents' house, had now returned to his mother's apartment.

"My father would not speak to him," Brandy said.

"Why?"

"Why? Because my father is a jerk!" She pronounced the word "jerk" in a loud tone with evident relish.

"Is your father speaking to you?" I asked.

Brandy answered in the negative and again explained this by exclaiming that her father was a "real jerk."

I turn to Brandy's mother to see her reaction and saw, to my amazement, a sympathetic and supportive maternal smile for her daughter on her face.

Trying to establish a bridge of common social values, I noted to Brandy that had she known her life would become so complicated, she probably would never have become pregnant at such an early age.

Like many other teenage mothers of whom I have asked this question, Brandy did not immediately answer. "No," she eventually said in a resolute manner, "I do not mind having the baby at all."

"Really?" I asked.

"I wanted it!" replied Brandy with defiance.

"But why?" I responded.

"Because I don't want to be an old woman when my children are grown up. Right, ma?" she finished, looking at her mother.

"That's right. I was sixteen when I got pregnant with her and eighteen with my second child. It worked out really good for me!" Matilda confirmed her daughter's "mature" decision, a decision of the kind that costs the taxpayers about $16 billion annually.

Unconquered, I undertook my last attempt to match my social values with Brandy's. "It's a pity you can't attend your regular school; you probably miss your friends a lot."

"No. I'm going to a special school," retorted Brandy. She pronounced the word "special" as if she were attending an Ivy League college.

"Is it really good?" I inquired naively.

With pride and determination in her voice, Brandy instructed me, "We study three hours a day there!"

"What about homework?"

"Homework!" Brandy stated incredulously. "No, we girls don't have time for *that*!"

As she and her mother were leaving the examining room, I realized that if I can manage to stay in practice a bit longer, in twelve or thirteen years I may see Matilda become a great-grandmother in her early forties and Brandy become a grandmother in her late twenties. Sixteen plus twelve equals twenty eight—true?

Soon after this visit Brandy became a mother. She was neither better nor worse than the average teenage mother in my practice.

At the age of one month, her baby, Brian, was brought to my office for an exam by Matilda because Brandy was at school. Brian was well fed and clothed and was developing normally, to our common pleasure.

"How is your daughter getting along with Willard?" I asked. "Oh, don't ask me," replied Matilda. "They are constantly arguing and fighting, behaving like kids. Maybe the reason for it is that Willard is smoking a lot of pot. Plus, after you have a baby, women develop PMS you know," Matilda enlightened me, "and Brandy has a lot of it."

At the age of two months, Brian was brought to the office by his mother for a cold, a runny nose, and general irritability. Brandy and Brian came two hours late for the appointment, as they had been unable to get a ride.

Eventually Willard drove them to my office. Willard was pacing back and forth in the exam room like a caged animal as Brandy "unpacked" Brian. To spite Willard, I suppose, Brandy told me that while Willard used to be her boyfriend, he was now only "a friend." Willard did not like this demotion in his standing. He kept himself under control, but I saw a malicious look in his eyes.

Fortunately Brian had only a mild infection, and there was no need for the dramatic measures that are sometime necessary in such a young child. After the result of a test I had done was available, I returned to the exam room where Brian had just recycled all his food through his quickly developing body. Brandy was cleaning her and Willard's child as do millions of mothers and fathers the world over, ignoring the thick, unpleasant smell.

"Well, well," was all I could say while observing this action which is so familiar to me and which is an inseparable part of being a parent.

At this moment Willard's face lit up as if he had thought of a great joke. "You stink even worse than him," he said in a teasing and contemptuous voice to Brandy— the mother of his child.

AND THE SHIP SAILS

SEVERAL YEARS ago, a fifteen-year-old mother, Brenda Walsh, brought her baby to be treated for a viral infection. The baby became sick on a weekend, and my office was closed, so I told Brenda to bring Cliff to the outpatient department of Doctors' Community Hospital, where he had been born the previous month.

The visit turned out to be quite exhausting. Cliff's examination did not elicit anything more abnormal than a stuffy nose, but Brenda was so passive and difficult to communicate with that I worried about the negative effect this could have on her child's health and development. I decided to watch this case closely before reporting it to social service.

Exhausted, I finally left the examining room. Unaware that the reception area of the outpatient department was separated from the waiting room by only a temporary, thin partition, I shared my concern about Brenda's apparent lack of interest in her child's condition with a nurse.

I had not mentioned Brenda by name, but before I finished speaking, a woman in her late forties flew into the reception area. Her face was twisted with anger, and she began screaming about how inappropriate my behavior was. This woman was Brenda's mother, Genine Lake, who had, unfortunately, overheard my innocent remark and was outraged. It was obvious to me that Mrs. Lake, was upset because she knew I was right about her daughter. Usually a grandmother wants to be in the exam room when a grandchild is examined, but Genine had not joined Brenda and her child. Perhaps, she wanted to let Brenda handle this necessary experience in the rearing of her child.

Though I had not broken any confidentiality, and had made my remark with the best of intentions, I would not have discussed anything about professional matters if I were aware it could be overheard by office visitors.

I was trying to explain the situation to Genine, but she was becoming more and more irate. Eventually, after a long conversation, she relented. We parted in peace.

After that encounter in the outpatient department, it was usually Genine who brought Cliff to my office for checkups. As I had expected, she provided very reliable care to her grandchild. Brenda rarely brought her child for visits. When she did, she was usually accompanied by her boyfriend, Russ, who wore lots of gold jewelry on his neck and hands and carried not one but two pagers on his belt.

The couple complained that Genine monopolized Cliff's care and was too strict with him. These conflicts occurred frequently, but I tried not to get involved in them.

Exactly a year and a half later, Brenda gave birth to another child, a girl, Sherry. Genine categorically refused to take care of this newborn baby. Brenda and her boyfriend, who brought their daughter in for her office visits, continued to criticize Genine for her many different shortcomings—their main complaint seemed to be Genine's insistence that Brenda marry her boyfriend.

Soon after Sherry's birth, the couple decided to move, along with their children, to Florida. I did not hear anything from them, but, two years later, Genine appeared at my office with three grandchildren. Brenda had given birth to another boy, Dexter, who was ten months old at the time of this visit. This child was by a different boyfriend Brenda had met while living in Florida.

Brenda had come back to the area, staying at her mother's house until she could find an apartment of her own. I was on vacation when Genine brought the children to the office so my partner examined Dexter. He was so dismayed by the child's slow development and by Genine's report of her daughter's parenting that he contacted the Department of Children and Family Services. Some changes did occur after this, but nothing dramatic enough to turn the situation around. The children still lived sometimes with their mother and sometimes with their grandmother, and they had very little stability in their lives. Luckily, my relations with both Genine and her daughter remained quite good.

The family again disappeared for a year. The next time I saw them, it was once again Genine who brought the three children in to see me. Genine had not changed at all in appearance—she was still very agile and had an animated expression on her small, narrow face. We hugged each other like old friends after a long parting. Genine was dressed not only neatly but with real elegance. Beautiful ruby stones decorated her jewelry. Her hair was elaborately done, with little golden cufflinks around every braid.

As we talked about past events, the children ran around my office in all directions, ignoring us and each other. Remembering my unpleasant lesson from the past, I was careful in my choice of words as I tried to establish some semblance of order in the examining room, but I soon realized that, far from objecting to my attempt to discipline her grandchildren, Genine was actually pleased to observe my success at the job of disciplinarian.

Finally, once order was established, I began to ask her about her daughter, Brenda.

"Ah," she sighed, "things are not very good."

"Drugs? Alcohol?" I asked in a low voice so that the children would not hear my question.

Genine answered in her regular voice, without heed to her grandchildren, "That and a lot more. I hardly see her. She comes and then disappears again with all her children." Gesturing toward her grandchildren, she sighed again. "I wish it were better. Cliff is not good. He is spoiled rotten and doesn't listen at all. I'm sick and tired of it. The others are not as bad, but I cannot discipline them; whatever I try to do is undone by Brenda and her current boyfriend. I hardly see them."

Mrs. Lake gave this information in a voice devoid of emotion. She was just enumerating sad facts of life. In her situation it would be dangerous for her to become emotional.

"Tell me something good, Genine. Does Brenda still live with Dexter's father?"

"No, no. This one left a lo-o-o-ong time ago."

Genine sighed again and, as before, with no outward sign of emotion, continued. "Two months ago, Brenda gave birth to her fourth child; this time she didn't tell me who the father was. She didn't go to the doctor when she was pregnant, although she had a medical card. The baby was born prematurely at University Hospital in Milwaukee and weighed less than two pounds. He had a lot of problems and is still in the hospital. He was too small and sick to be transferred to Chicago."

Then, as if brushing all this sadness away, Genine smiled and, in an optimistic tone of voice, continued. "But, recently, my new grandson, Clarence, is doing really well. The doctors at the hospital say he is going to be discharged in a couple of days. So you are going to see the baby and Brenda." She paused and added, "Unless Brenda takes all the children and goes off somewhere with one of her friends."

After the visit we shook hands warmly. Genine gave me a big smile, and I could see sparkles in her eyes. She was not beaten down by her daughter's lifestyle. Though she was somewhat critical of her grandchildren and disturbed by her daughter's behavior, Genine was not willing to give up on her desire to live a happy life. She was fully resolved to live such a life regardless of her daughter's decisions.

LIBERATED COUPLES

IF NOT for the public aid insurance that covered Eunice Groppy and her daughter, I would have thought that Eunice and the child's father belonged to middle-class America. The parents were not married, and both were nineteen. Their child almost shone; she was wearing a beautiful and expensive dress and was peacefully sucking on a pacifier.

Both parents were so incredibly compatible that I had a hard time resisting the logical question that comes up in such a situation. I realized, however, that if I asked why they hadn't gotten married, I had only a very small chance of hearing the full truth; one of the main reasons could be their desire to continue receiving welfare benefits.

All I could say was that I was so impressed with their wonderful relationship that I wished I saw a wedding ring on Eunice's hand. Eunice sighed, "We don't even have the money for a good ring."

"If you really promise me that you are going to get married," I offered semijokingly, "I will pitch in for a ring and take you and your baby straight from here to the closest available minister."

To the laughter of everyone who was present in the room, except, of course, the baby, the father answered, "There is no need to do that; my own father is a minister."

I observed another example of the modern, devil-may-care attitude, that prevails over the institution of marriage when Bernice Gladley, a warm and caring eighteen-year-old mother, brought her one-year-old girl in for a regular checkup. From the day her daughter was born, Bernice was on welfare. She now lived with her boy friend and their child at her grandparents' house in a suburb of Chicago.

"Don't you think that for your child's benefit it would be better if you got married?" I asked Bernice as I looked at her pretty little daughter.

"I don't think so," answered Bernice sincerely and, sharing her rich life experience with me, explained, "What difference would it make? My daughter sees him every day anyway."

A PIMPLE

IT WAS not difficult for me to guess the reason for this visit when I saw the face of Arnice Wild's mother. Mrs. Wild was a nurse at a large hospital; she had accompanied her seventeen-year-old daughter to the office on this visit. Arnice's reaction also was not unusual, though it was obvious that she was very embarrassed. She had a forced laugh and tried to act as if she had no reason at all to be in a doctor's office.

As I had expected, I heard the familiar request from Arnice's mother, "Doctor, I would like to find out if my daughter is pregnant."

I asked Arnice when she had her last menstrual period. She replied that to the best of her knowledge it had been three months ago. Her mother angrily scolded Arnice for not telling her sooner. Arnice took the Fifth.

To verify the diagnosis, blood was taken for a pregnancy test after I examined Arnice. "My boyfriend wants me to have the baby," Arnice informed both her mother and me while I drew the blood for the test.

"And what about you?" I asked her innocently.

"I don't mind," answered Arnice with a coquettish smile on her face, as she became even more embarrassed. I praised her for her courageous behavior during the procedure, gave her the lollipop she had asked for, and was ready to leave the exam room.

As I stood up to leave the exam room, I heard Arnice's voice. "May I ask you a question?" she said while sucking on the lollipop.

"Of course," I replied.

Arnice pointed to a tiny eruption on her smooth and tender cheek and asked me with nervous apprehension, "Doctor, what can I do with this pimple?"

I tried, unsuccessfully, to conceal the paternal tone which crept into my voice, "Arnice, we are worrying about your future and here you are fretting about a small pimple."

"But Doc," replied Arnice, slightly annoyed, "I had this pimple before I got pregnant!"

IN PURSUIT OF ACADEMIC EXCELLENCE

IF NOT for the experience and knowledge accumulated by me during my five decades of life, I might begin to believe that it is I who have lost touch with reality and live in a world of illusion.

Though some of Deanna Fountain's views about life do coincide with mine, overall our basic values are so different and we are so far apart from one another, that I cannot even argue with her.

Deanna, a seventeen-year-old with an above average intelligence, took life very seriously. She had just given birth to a wonderful, eight-pound baby girl at the local hospital. Though we had never met before, our conversation was friendly and earnest.

Deanna's health care was covered by her parents' insurance, and her child was going to be insured by the Department of Public Aid. Her parents were blue-collar workers who had two other children, also girls. The sisters were older than Deanna, had graduated from college, and were both working in the publishing business—one was an editor, the other an administrator. Both were divorced.

Deanna told me that her parents were going to help her raise the baby. Her main preoccupation was school; she did not want her responsibilities as a mother to interfere with her schoolwork.

Deanna presented the epitome of youth. Though she had given birth only twelve hours earlier, she looked ready to give a pom-pom-girl performance. Her face was round with dark eyes, and her skin was smooth and unblemished. She had a frequent smile on her pretty face.

Not many teenage mothers are as intelligent and willing to share their thoughts as Deanna was, so I, trying to enrich my professional experience, began asking her questions about her life.

In olden times, usually the young mother was left by the father of the newborn child. Not these days. From many women and, indeed, from Deanna, I hear that usually it is the mother who decides against marriage to the father of their child. I was interested to know from Deanna why she wouldn't even consider the possibility of marriage to the baby's father. Though Deanna was not eager to answer, I repeated the question.

"Well, at our young age relationships do not usually come to anything serious. To tell you the truth, all he was able to do well at his age was to show his physical love for me. Otherwise, he's not mature enough and isn't interested in anything but having a good time."

Once Deanna had become pregnant and had told her family of it, she transferred to a school for pregnant students, which she found to be better than the one she had previously attended.

The school was located in downtown Chicago. In order to get there, Deanna, who lived in a northern suburb of Chicago, took the city bus. For a while she was unable to make these trips because she suffered from uterine contractions, a consequence, she had been told by her obstetrician, of a chlamydia infection. During this period a special tutor from the school system came to her home all the way from downtown Chicago in order to prevent her from lagging behind in her schoolwork.

Naturally, Deanna's obstetrician told her that chlamydia is a sexually transmitted disease. Apparently the boyfriend she thought was so in love with her was not limiting his loving propensities to her only.

Deanna was expecting Ervin, her boyfriend, to arrive soon with flowers. The reason that he hadn't yet been by, she told me, was that she had gone to the hospital several times with false labor, so this time Ervin had again thought that the pains were not real.

"Seeing how responsibly you take your life, Deanna," I said, "I am really surprised that such an intelligent girl like you was not careful enough to use the Pill."

"I don't know why I didn't use the Pill, but he did use condoms. Two times." Deanna looked so young and innocent that I was reluctant to ask her how many times her boyfriend should have used a condom. Instead, I again asked her why she hadn't prevented this pregnancy. Deanna thought for a moment and then blurted out "Maybe I should have been more responsible."

"Indeed, Deanna," I thought.

The last time I saw Deanna's child was when he was eleven months old. As I had expected, her parents were helping her to be a good mother, and she continued to be a good student. Sometimes Ervin came into my office with Deanna and the baby, but the couple are not planning to get married anytime in the foreseeable future. Maybe one of these days.

A COMPLICATED CASE OF CONSTIPATION

AN EARLY morning phone call woke me up. It was Maureen on the line, a nurse from the local hospital's newborn nursery who has known me for many years. In spite of the difficulties of her job, Maureen was able to retain a sense of humor all day.

"Good morning, Dr. Vladimir," she said. "Congratulations! You have a wonderful newborn, a baby girl, a lovely child weighing in at more than seven pounds. A sheer delight. The mother is so surprised she had a baby she still has a hard time believing that the baby is her own."

I examined Mollie's child a short while later, a beautiful, healthy baby with a pleasant appearance. Mollie Moore was a patient of mine, a fourteen-year-old teenager. Mollie was an average child from a white-collar family. She was pleasant and friendly. Like any adolescent child she visited my office rather infrequently—once or twice a year at most.

With an ironic smile Maureen told me the more complete story. The day before the baby was born, at around 9:30 in the evening, Mollie began complaining of stomach pains. After talking with her parents, it was decided that the most probable reason for these pains was constipation—Mollie had not had a bowel movement for two or three days. The enema they gave Mollie did not produce the expected effect; her pains were getting worse. Along with her mother and her fourteen-year-old boyfriend, Mollie came to the emergency room, where, to her disappointment, she was told by Dr. Clifford that the reason for her indisposition was not constipation but a full-term pregnancy.

As I later learned, Mollie never once had thought she was pregnant; as for the enlarged size of her stomach, she had explained this to herself as an indication that she was growing and becoming more mature. She hid her growing stomach from other people and from herself by wearing loose-fitting tops over baggy jeans. As for being concerned about her lack of menstrual periods, Mollie was not going to try to penetrate the secrets of nature. Nature knew best. To distract herself from paying too much attention to the disquieting changes in her body, she got busy discovering the joys of sex with her boyfriend, Abe. She had at least four things in common with Abe: they were in the same class; they were well-behaved students; sex education was their favorite subject; and they liked to chew gum.

When I entered Mollie's room to tell the family about the newborn, I found Mollie with her mother, Carol, and her boyfriend, a tall, lean adolescent. His face had never known the touch of a razor, and only the acne on his forehead testified to his budding sexual development.

My good news about this new member of the family did not produce the expected response—Mollie was looking at an invisible spot on the ceiling, while Abe, the baby's alleged father, concentrated intently on a game, a one-player tournament he played on a pocket Nintendo machine as he chewed a huge wad of gum.

Only Carol looked at me when I concluded my pleasant report. There was not a hint of satisfaction on her face even after she heard the good news. "Doctor, a moment ago Mollie came to an important decision in her life," Carol said after a small pause.

"What kind of important decision?" I addressed my question to Mollie but her mother answered for her. "Doctor, we have decided that the baby will go up for adoption. None of us," Carol pointed her finger toward Mollie, Abe, and then herself, "none of us are ready for this baby; she just was not planned at all.

"Therefore, just before you came in, we called an adoption agency, and they told us that the baby had an opportunity to be adopted right away. There are a lot of childless couples around who would be very happy to have my grandchild. This will be a good deed that my daughter can perform in her youth.

"It was smart of Mollie to refuse to touch the baby or even to take a peek at her in the delivery room to avoid bonding. Mollie made a mistake, but now she is behaving like a responsible, mature person."

Carol was so persuasive in her speech that I wished she could have been present during the intercourse that had occurred between her daughter and Abe so that then, at the critical moments, she would have been able to help the adolescents with her wise advice.

"Mollie was very upset," Carol continued, "when, instead of constipation as she had thought, Dr. Clifford told her in the emergency room, without any sensitivity to her feelings, I might add, that she was pregnant. She wasn't pleased with this news at all.

"I never thought that Mollie was pregnant," continued Carol, as if she were anticipating my question. "Of course I could not miss that she was getting bigger, but you know my family—we are all predisposed to obesity, even our cat is fat—so I thought that Mollie was just following in our footsteps. Besides, she recently started to eat a lot of ice cream; she was like addicted to it."

At this moment I heard many beeps, followed by the ringing, victorious voice of the newborn baby's father. "I won, I won," he exclaimed as he tightly held in his sweaty, narrow hands his security blanket—the pocket Nintendo game.

Mollie did not react to her mother's monologue or to her boyfriend's exultation over his manual dexterity; she was depressed and unwilling to talk. I did not want to bother her and was going to leave the room when Carol, who apparently felt more relaxed and less inhibited, decided to ask me a professional question.

"Doctor," she said confidentially, "my daughter Ellen, she's a year older than Mollie, has also recently had problems with her bowel movements. Her boyfriend has been hanging around her all the time. Can she come to your office tomorrow for a pregnancy test? I would rather be safe than sorry."

Carol paused for a second and had a second thought. "Never mind," she concluded. "Before she comes to you, let me give her a good enema."

IT'S CHILDREN, STUPID

ONE OF the things that helped Bill Clinton beat George Bush in the 1992 presidential campaign was a sign Clinton supporters carried that read, "It's the economy, stupid."

I remembered this saying after Grizelda Saldivar's second visit to my office. Grizelda was a beautiful and healthy former patient of mine. She had grown up in a stable, middle-class family. Grizelda's mother was a friendly and polite woman. At the time of this visit Grizelda was seventeen years old; I had last seen her three years earlier and recently had received a call from her mother, who asked me in a dispassionate but polite voice whether I would be willing to treat Grizelda's child, a child born out of wedlock. Grizelda was living on her own and had public aid insurance. I told Mrs. Saldivar that we would welcome her granddaughter in our office.

A week or two later, I had the pleasure of examining Grizelda's daughter, little Alisa, who was only one month old at the time.

Grizelda was a tall, well-built, beautiful brunette with an elaborate tattoo on her right hand. She was very natural in her role as a single parent—a frequent feature among teenage mothers. The modern teenage mothers, from my observation, do not see themselves abandoned and deceived, as they are frequently portrayed. For them, being a single parent is an accepted societal norm. Grizelda looked very happy, as did her precious and charming daughter.

Grizelda was not usually a talkative person, and only my position as her child's pediatrician made her more willing to talk about issues other than those that personally interested her.

My first question was very naive from her point of view. When, with an almost trembling voice, I asked her whether she had wanted to have this baby, she gave me such a strong "Yes", that, for a moment, I lost my nerve in interviewing her. But I could not give up and was compelled for professional reasons to ask about her boyfriend.

"I don't have a boyfriend." Grizelda cut me off immediately.

"But the baby had a father. For medical reasons I need to know about him," I replied.

After some hesitation, Grizelda told me that Alisa's father was an adolescent who had seen his child only once. He had a serious drug abuse problem and was going to marry some other girl soon.

She then told me with the pride of a truly independent person that she was getting a $280 check from Public Aid each month.

"Good for you. But what would you do if this money became unavailable?"

"Then I would live with my parents," Grizelda said as if surprised by my simplicity.

She shared an apartment with a seventeen-year-old girlfriend who, as I found out a couple of months later, also had a child, although that child was living with her parents. Both women paid only utilities, as this house was owned by Grizelda's grandmother.

"I suppose your mother was upset when you told her that you were pregnant?" I said, making an educated guess.

Grizelda spoke as if she were the representative of a generation that sees new horizons unknown to the older people. "At first, yes. For a while she was nervous about it, but later she calmed down." Then, with a patronizing air of superiority that showed how critical she was of her mother's reactionary views, she added, "She'd better learn how to accept it."

Grizelda came for her child's next appointment with her mother. Mrs. Saldivar, whom Grizelda was patiently coaching on how to take care of Alisa, took Grizelda's bossing with silent dignity.

The visit was coming to an end. Mrs. Saldivar took Alisa out of the office while Grizelda, waited for me to complete a note in the baby's chart.

"Grizelda," I said getting ready to leave the examining room, "I was quite impressed with your decisions the last time I saw you. I have a couple of questions I'd like to ask you that I don't want to ask in your mother's presence."

Grizelda looked at me with mild curiosity.

"Ok. What's the question?" replied she looking at me with her beautiful velvet brown eyes.

"You know, I am so intrigued; did you really want this baby at your young age and with no husband?"

Grizelda gave me an aristocratic, supercilious smile and again confirmed her decision with a strong "Yes!"

I began to doubt that I should ask these questions and take up Grizelda's valuable time, but the desire to understand the psychology of the younger generation overtook me, "What about your boyfriend? Did he also want to become a father?"

"Yes!" Grizelda said with impatience.

Risking the loss of Grizelda's respect by appearing to be a person who does not comprehend people and their decisions, I said, "Sure, he wanted you to have the baby, but once the baby was born, he disappeared."

Grizelda's face showed her astonishment with my naiveté. "He wanted to have a baby, but he did not want to stay with me," Grizelda said, reminding me of a strict teacher from my grammar school.

Grizelda began to show signs of restlessness; obviously, from her standpoint, she was annoyed with my backwardness.

"Grizelda, please, one more question. You did not tell me—why did you want to become pregnant?"

Grizelda looked at me as I had just fallen from the moon. Looking down at me, she let me know what a simpleton she thought me to be, "Because I like babies, that's why!"

How inconsiderate of me, even how stupid of me not to understand such a simple thing.

NOT ONLY DOCTORS ARE PAGED

IT WAS 10 p.m., and I had still not finished my working day which had begun at 6 a.m. Luckily for me this does not happen too frequently. The admission of two-month-old B. J. Colby was the reason for my presence in the hospital emergency room at this late hour.

B. J. was admitted to the hospital because of a very high fever, 103°F. Current thinking in pediatric medicine is that when a very young baby (up to two to three months old) runs a high fever and exhibits no obvious causal source of infection, the fever is considered to be "guilty until proven otherwise": experience has shown that these fevers might precede such serious conditions as sepsis or meningitis, conditions that can be confirmed or disproved only with lab tests. Until the results of these tests are available, the baby should receive large doses of antibiotics for at least forty eight hours on the presumption that it could be a serious illness.

I had never treated baby Colby before, he was referred to our group because we were on call for pediatric service at the hospital this night. The baby was brought to the ER by his mother, eighteen-year-old Sharon Colby, and his father, twenty-one-year-old Dave Fisher. Dave wore the badges of the local culture: two thick golden earrings and a pager on his belt. The latter provided for the former.

Sharon was very nervous, questioned any procedure I suggested, and, when it came time to perform a spinal tap, became hysterical. It took a long talk to persuade her to give her permission for this procedure, in which a specimen of the fluid that fills the cavity of the brain and spine is taken by inserting a needle into the midline area of the lower back. When Sharon's fears came to a boiling point, she asked to speak to her boyfriend and asked a nurse to call him in from outside—he was out there as he was a chain-smoker.

Despite her young age, Sharon looked at least eight years older than she was—the result, no doubt, of her unhealthy lifestyle and her use of drugs and alcohol. Nevertheless, she was still able to function adequately, and her baby did not look neglected or abused. He was well nourished and dressed in nice clothing.

The necessary tests were finally performed, the treatment was initiated, and the baby was ready to be transferred from the ER to the pediatric ward. To my surprise and relief, Ms. Colby had completely changed her attitude: she looked docile and satisfied. At last we had a normal conversation while I explained my plan of treatment to her. I then asked her whether she was going to stay with the baby. She answered affirmatively.

In conclusion I told Ms. Colby that I was going upstairs to the pediatric floor in order to make sure that the nurse in charge understood my instructions. She nodded her head in acknowledgment and then said solemnly, in a hoarse voice, "Make sure they have a good room and a bed for us."

I promised to look into her request and directed my steps to the pediatric floor.

To be on time to my office for the scheduled appointments of the day, I left home the next day for rounds at a very early time, around 6:30 a.m. By 7 a.m. I was already on the pediatric floor ready to start my morning rounds. I was happy to hear from the night nurse that the baby's condition had gotten a little bit better since his admission. Moreover, his temperature, the main reason for his admission, was normal.

With a chart and a couple of instruments in hand, I entered the patient's room with the nurse. To my surprise I perceived in the scantily lit hospital room the thick smell of alcohol. Trying to find the light switch, I moved around the room by sense of touch until I was able to turn on the lights. In the crib B. J. was sleeping peacefully. A green light blinked reassuringly on the system that monitored the IV that was providing him with fluids and antibiotics.

I looked into the bed that stood close to B. J.'s crib. What did I see on this bed! There, in a haze of alcohol vapors, lay Ms. Colby and her boyfriend, locked in a tight, inseparable embrace.

What a fool I am! How could I have failed to understand? When Sharon had emphatically requested "a good room and a bed for us," she had obviously included in the pronoun "us" her boyfriend. I should have realized.

Before I was able to speak, a pager came on, breaking the silence in the room. It was not mine; someone was looking for Dave Fisher, who was still sleeping soundly at this early hour.

10

DESTROYING BODIES, POLLUTING MINDS, LOSING LIVES

The epidemic of drug and alcohol abuse in the United States, which began in the mid-1960s, is continuing to take its toll on millions of Americans of all ages. Sloganeering such as "Say 'No' to Drugs", and "A Drug-Free America", have not, as could easily have been predicted, effected any appreciable change in the progressively worsening course of this epidemic; perhaps it has given some temporary peace of mind to people who invent or love slogans or to those people who are caught up in wishful thinking.

The reason that the slogans and numerous, enthusiastic antidrug movements are failing is not that those who become "hooked" on drugs lack the knowledge that they should "Say 'No' to Drugs"—as a matter of fact, many of these people are quite intelligent. The problem is that their general psychological orientation is not conducive to constructive behavior; for many reasons they are choosing a destructive lifestyle, of which drug and alcohol abuse is only a part.

In addition, the ongoing and systematic destruction of our society's traditional family structure and values makes the pursuit of a productive and meaningful life less desirable for some than is the pursuit of immediate gratification and an escape from reality.

It is a pity that people are universally worried about the soulless environment (which has to be protected as well) but are seemingly unconcerned in the face of the systematic pollution and destruction of the minds of their fellow human beings. A sizable group among several millions of Americans who have a drug problem, consists of adolescents. It looks as if our environment will probably survive the abuse perpetrated by the human race, but people, living people, adolescents, children, and now, even newborns, are losing their only chance at life to chemicals that are polluting the environment of their bodies.

One example of the outrageous misunderstandings that abound on what the proliferation of drugs will mean to the future of our culture stands out: some practical people, as they call themselves, insist that the best way to win the war on drugs is to stop waging it. Legalize drugs, they say, open up Pandora's box, let addicts have their drugs for as long as they can pay for them. These people overlook the fact that this would transform our world into a stage for social Darwinism: naturally, the fittest may survive, but what about the weak? What if the weak individual happens to be your son or daughter? Shall we sacrifice one, two, or more generations of people trying to prove the obvious fact that drugs have a devastating effect on the lives and minds of those who take them?

One rationale for the appeal to legalize drugs is economic. But can we transfer the language of money into the price of a human life lost to drugs? Would those who propose to legalize drugs for other people also be willing to apply this to their own children? Are they ready to put a price on their own child's life? Are we still Homo sapiens with hearts of humans, or have we became Homo economicus?

Drug and alcohol addiction is one of the movements of mankind toward self-destruction; sometimes the devastation of addiction is immediate, and sometimes it takes a longer period of time. The blind application of the dogma of freedom of choice ignores the fact that this choice was formulated not for people to whom freedom meant the right to be destructive, but for people to whom freedom meant the right to lead a productive life. What freedom of choice is being offered to the children born to mothers who have exercised their freedom to use cocaine during pregnancy? These children, each of whom is an individual with human rights equal to the rights of their mothers, have no freedom of choice during the first, most critical nine months of their development, their life in utero. During this period so critical for their future, their mother's blood provides them not only with life-sustaining fluids but also with toxic substances that frequently affect their developing brain irreversibly.

The following stories are not intended to be a social prescription; rather, my purpose is to share some of my encounters with real flesh-and-blood people—both adults and children—who were born for joy and happiness but, instead, encountered a powerful enemy on the path of life: the destructive effects of alcohol and psychotropic drugs. Some of these victims were able to survive—some were not so lucky.

A CHILD PROTECTION INVESTIGATOR

THE FIRST time I saw her, Pamela Rivers, a twenty-five-year-old woman, looked horrible despite her young age. Looking at her then, I wondered how long it had been since a smile had brightened her face. Of all the features of her depersonalized appearance, only her eyes, with their anxious stare, remained alert.

Pamela already had one child—a four-year-old boy. She had given birth to her second child, a full-term baby, by cesarean section the day before our meeting. This infant's weight was far below the norm for a baby carried to term. The reason for the baby's low birth weight was intrauterine growth retardation—the result of Ms. Rivers's drug abuse and heavy smoking during her pregnancy.

Both of Ms. Rivers's boyfriends were claiming to be the baby's father. From Pamela's standpoint the father was boyfriend #1; but boyfriend #2, from whom Pamela was estranged at the time, claimed to be the real McCoy. Ms. Rivers had not come to a final decision about whose name her newborn baby was going to take. Meanwhile, Pamela's boyfriends had been involved in two bloody fistfights in her room, both of which had been quickly stopped by the security guards. After the second fight, the would-be fathers were forbidden to visit Pamela in the hospital.

Ms. Rivers had been on welfare, and, therefore, her medical expenses would have been fully covered by the state, but she had not made a single visit to a physician during her pregnancy. Upon her admission to the hospital, she freely admitted to her regular use of drugs. Her drug of choice was crack cocaine. Not only did her urine contain cocaine, but the urine of her newborn baby contained it as well.

To my surprise, by the fourth day after her delivery, Ms. Rivers's appearance had dramatically changed for the better: the hospital environment, with its poor accessibility to illegal drugs, had transformed her into a nice looking, even an attractive, woman.

At this time I had a chance to have a friendly talk with Pamela. "Ms. Rivers, you are on your way to losing your life to drugs," I said to her. "You put your life and the life of your newborn child in serious jeopardy. Even immediately before the baby was born you were using cocaine. Why?"

"I'm not responsible for that, Doctor. My boyfriend brought me some crack and talked me into taking it to celebrate July 4." Ms. Rivers voiced this explanation to me with no trace of humor in her voice.

"Do you realize, Ms. Rivers, how bad it was that you were doing drugs during your pregnancy? For God's sake, why did you use cocaine before your baby was born?" I asked this question out of desperation. Feeling helpless in the face of the evil in the world, I expected no answer from Ms. Rivers.

Suddenly, I noticed an ironic smile on Ms. Rivers's face. An awakened intelligence glowed from her. "I should be able to give you a better answer than most people," she said. "My mother, who died a year ago, worked for the Department of Children and Family Services as a social worker. And," she finished with a sigh, "until last year I worked for DCFS as a child protection investigator."

Though Ms. Rivers seemed sincere, it was difficult for me to believe her; she read this on my face. With the same bitter smile, she took the purse that lay next to her, dug out an old ID, and handed it to me. I saw there the picture of a gentle, tender, merry woman's face— the face that Ms. Rivers had worn only one and one half years earlier.

ANOTHER ORDINARY CASE

MOTHERS WHO use drugs by no means stop loving and caring about their children—they simply reach a limit beyond which they are unable to function as parents. Many of these mothers are warm, intelligent, and even sensitive individuals. I have observed great love and devotion to children even in families where the mother was on the brink of ceasing to function as an independent person. These parents' first priority, however—their children—gradually becomes overshadowed by the deep psychological problems that are exacerbated by the effects of drugs on the body and mind. Due to the destructive action of drugs, not only do these parents lose control over their children's upbringing, they lose control over their own destiny as well. To use a medical analogy, drug addiction can be characterized as a cancer in the body of the family. The metastasis of such a cancer can affect any member of a family, bringing disease, misery, and death.

Ms. Ammer still looked Ok, although she had been using cocaine for three years. Her nervous, anxious manner, abrupt motions, and unhealthy appearance, however, betrayed to an experienced observer that she was drug-dependent.

Ms. Ammer had visited an obstetrician only once or twice during her pregnancy.

During our first meeting, Ms. Ammer—after the toxicologic screening had established the presence of cocaine, marijuana, and alcohol in her urine—admitted that she "did" drugs two or three times a week, mostly on weekends. Like many other women I have spoken to about a drug problem, she blamed her habit on her boyfriend. While she never specified the particular method he used to persuade her to intoxicate her mind and body, she stated that he had "turned her on" to taking drugs.

Ms. Ammer eagerly agreed with me that she was doing the wrong thing by using alcohol and drugs, especially during the time when she was pregnant with her baby. When, however, I asked her if she was ready to make a genuine commitment to stop using drugs, she answered that she was not ready for such "a difficult decision" and needed more time to think it over.

The following day the toxicological screening of Ms. Ammer's newborn daughter established the presence of cocaine in the baby's urine as well, and this automatically started a DCFS investigation. Four days later the case went to the court. The judge, taking into account that it was the first offense, allowed Ms. Ammer to keep the newborn baby in her home. For the first months of the infant's life a public health nurse would monitor the baby's condition. If, during this period, there were no obvious signs of neglect or abuse by the parent, the surveillance of Ms. Ammer's family would gradually cease.

Obviously, the assumption on the part of DCFS and the judicial system is that mothers like Ms. Ammer will gradually stop using drugs. Like so many other hopeful expectations, that is hardly likely to happen. Thus, Ms. Ammer's child is destined, from her first days of life, to join the burgeoning number of American children who are growing up in families in which self-destruction by self-intoxication is common—not the ideal environment for providing good role models.

A LESSON IN ARITHMETIC

EVEN THOUGH I had known Herman Jefferson ten years ever since the birth of his only son, Armando, and even though his son visited our office so frequently that his health record was twice as large as that of an average child of his age, I could not say very much about Herman. His appearance, however, was easy to describe: he was in his early thirties, rather tall and well built, with a sharp-featured, clean-shaven face. His eyes were blue and deep set. He had thick, blond and curly hair.

Herman's wife died in a car accident when Armando was almost two years old. Since his wife's death Herman together with his parents was taking care of Armando. Though Herman was always tense, he by no means ever produced the impression of a father who did not do his best for his child. To the contrary: on more than one occasion, I had told him that he could save himself the trouble of coming into the office by using over-the-counter remedies for common problems like a mild cold.

Herman and his son had much in common. Like his father, Armando was also tense and anxious. However, if Herman hardly ever smiled, Armando liked to laugh any time he was talking. This laughter was not natural but, instead, served as a way to release tension. As artificial and superficial as his laughter was, it was, nevertheless, musical and pleasant to the ear—and it was a part of Armando's personality.

For many years, Armando had been accompanied to the office only by his father, until a couple of years ago, when they disappeared from my office for around six months. The explanation I got at the time for Armando's absence was that the family had moved to another area for a short time. Herman had come in with his son twice since then. After that I did not see Herman in my office. Instead, Herman's mother, Mrs. Nicolette Jefferson, Armando's sixty-two-seven-year-old grandmother, brought Armando to the office.

It was so unusual for me not to see Herman with his son that, on Mrs. Jefferson's second visit to our office, I asked where Herman was.

"He is in a psychiatric hospital," Mrs. Jefferson answered abruptly, without enthusiasm, avoiding my gaze.

"Why is he there?" I asked her with sincere surprise. I would never have thought that Herman would need psychiatric treatment—nothing in his behavior or general appearance indicated it.

"He had a chemical imbalance." Mrs. Jefferson explained Herman's condition to me with this single sentence.

I was well aware that "chemical imbalance" is a commonly used euphemism for a drug problem. I also knew that, though Mrs. Jefferson's answer was brief, it might not be because she was untalkative. Frequently, people who ask about the condition of a loved one do not have the patience or interest to listen to the response; they ask only for the sake of propriety. Eventually, the one to whom these questions are addressed gets used to this lack of genuine interest and finds the best solution is to respond with the shortest possible answer.

However, simply by listening to the story of the victims of these unhappy situations, listening to their grief and despair about their difficult walk through life's ordeals, people who ask after a family member in trouble can show a token of human compassion to help their fellow human beings. Mrs. Jefferson, who saw my sincere interest in Herman's condition, gave me the details of her son's hospitalization. Herman had developed a condition that was close to a psychotic reaction after many years of systematic cocaine use.

Several years ago I would have been shocked to hear that someone like Herman could be involved with drugs, but, unfortunately, having seen so many similar cases, I realized with sadness that the story did not affect me as it once would have. I listened to Mrs. Jefferson with the unhappy and disturbing understanding of my own inability to help Herman help himself.

Mrs. Jefferson spoke in a soft, monotonous voice—a technique that people regularly use to avoid revealing their emotional involvement. She told me that Herman's wife desperately tried to pull him out of his addiction before she died.

Herman, who had worked for many years as an electrician, had recently begun having problems at work and had been told that if he did not improve, he would be fired. Unable to control his chronic cocaine addiction on his own, Herman entered the hospital for treatment.

I have noticed that children who belong to families where one or both parents are involved with drugs and alcohol are rarely protected from the traumatic knowledge of this drug use. Armando sat in the room but showed no reaction to Mrs. Jefferson's talk about Herman. Like many other times, my indication of Armando's presence resulted in his grandmother's sad explanation: "He knows all about it, none better."

Mrs. Jefferson was in a hurry, as she had to leave to go to her own doctor—she was not a young woman and had health problems of her own. At our parting, Mrs. Jefferson spoke in the soft monotone she used to hide the pain and misery she felt at her unsuccessful attempts to help her son.

We shook hands, and, to my surprise, she thanked me.

"For what?" I asked. "I can't see how I've helped you. I was just asking questions, that's all."

"At least you are asking questions," Mrs. Jefferson answered. "I have not had a chance to tell my story for a long time."

We met again three months later. Armando had abdominal pain. He handled himself in his usual manner, excitedly making comments and asking questions in his slightly stuttering, ringing voice and interrupting himself with his silvery, musical laugh. Frequently, the louder the child, the more emotional tension the child is trying to resolve.

If Armando's appearance was not affected by his father's affliction, his grandmother presented a different picture. No, by no means was Mrs. Jefferson close to a nervous breakdown. To protect herself from being broken by stress, she had escaped into a shell to shield herself from the reality of life. Tensions and troubles had warped her appearance and had prematurely drawn deep lines and wrinkles on her face, forming large bags under her eyes and ringing them with deep, dark circles.

Things were not going well with her son. Herman had gotten involved with bad crowd—people whose names Mrs. Jefferson did not even know. He had not been home for more than a month. Herman was in a disastrous situation, and his prognosis was very grave. His appearance had deteriorated drastically, he was "nonstop on cocaine," had quit his job, and was living on the money, that he borrowed from friends and relatives.

"I am losing hope for his future," Mrs. Jefferson continued. "I wish I had an idea of when my son would stop his wild despicable living."

"Well, you cannot do more than you are doing now," I remarked. "Look how fortunate it is that you are around. Isn't it great that you and your husband are able to take such good care of your grandchild? Do you have many grandchildren?"

I had obviously said something that Mrs. Jefferson wanted to hear and I saw how my words enlivened her face. A warm, maternal pride lighted up her tired eyes. "I have five grandchildren, Doctor," she answered. "In addition to Herman, I have three other children."

I then saw another Mrs. Jefferson, not the one I knew who was hiding from the world, but a woman who was proud and happy to tell about her life's achievements.

One son was vice president of a big bank, another son was an archeologist, and the younger daughter was a research physicist. "Only Herman did not make it. I don't know whose fault it was—he was such a promising child," Mrs. Jefferson concluded.

"Mrs. Jefferson, you should indeed feel proud of your children's successes. It only proves that what happened to Herman was not your fault. I see the mourning and misery on your face, and it is killing you. But Herman, only Herman, not anybody else, chose his course of self-destruction. You have to think about your own survival—you have your own soul and your own life. Have pity on yourself, Mrs. Jefferson. Your worries are literally killing you. Stop torturing yourself."

Mrs. Jefferson softly smiled to me. "Doctor, I have thought many times about what you are telling me now, but it has not entirely helped me to find a way out of my unhappiness. For me, my children are like four extremities of my body. So what if both legs and one arm are healthy and strong; the arm that is sore, swollen, and sick—does it hurt me less just because the other extremities do not bother me?

"I wish that three pluses and one minus equaled zero in the sum of my emotional well-being. Unfortunately, my life is not a lesson in arithmetic, and my heart is not a calculator. It's the heart of a human, and this heart hurts a lot."

A DEAL

ALFONSA CERVANTES, a twenty-three-year-old, mother of newborn twins admitted that she had been using cocaine when a nurse asked her some routine questions on admission to the hospital's Labor and Delivery Department. Mrs. Cervantes was a welfare recipient. She was married and already had a six-year-old son. At the time the twins were born, the family was unable to pay rent and was living in the apartment of Alfonsa's parents, who had come from Colombia years earlier. Alfonsa had a satisfactory record of prenatal visits.

Above average height, still young-looking, dressed in simple, attractive clothing, Alfonsa would have been indistinguishable from the other women in the maternity ward but for the subtle indications of her addiction to drugs. She had a sallow complexion and was irritable and untalkative. Her anxious eyes carefully avoided any eye contact. Alfonsa created a separation between herself and the outer world, producing the impression of a little animal that concealed itself in a safe underground burrow, communicating with the surrounding world only by sticking the tip of its nose out of its hideout.

Despite her avoidance of direct and open contact, Mrs. Cervantes asked me good questions about the care of her newborn babies. When I left the room, I was introduced to Mrs. Cervantes's parents—ordinary-looking people who spoke broken English. Their faces expressed a peculiar combination of joy and bitterness.

Two weeks after her discharge from the hospital, Alfonsa and her mother brought the newborn girls for a well-baby examination. At the appropriate moment, I told Mrs. Cervantes that I would be happy to perform my duties as a pediatrician to her lovely twins only if she promised to completely abstain from the use of illegal drugs.

"Is it a deal?" I concluded.

"Yes, it's a deal," Alfonsa answered and then added that it had been her own intention to quit taking drugs.

After that visit, Mrs. Cervantes and her children were regular visitors in the office. Judging by Alfonsa's appearance, I could see that even if she were deceiving me by continuing to do drugs, she was well adjusted and was competent to take care of her children.

Whenever I reminded Alfonsa of our deal, she did not protest but silently shook her curly head of hair from side to side to let me know that she was still faithful to her promise.

Two years passed. Mrs. Cervantes came to the office for a checkup for her children, who were, on this day, all dressed in bedazzling, Spanish-style outfits. Hardly a trace remained of the anxious, irritable woman Mrs. Cervantes had been when I first met her: her complexion was healthy, her eyes were clear, she moved with grace and energy.

"You know, Dr. Tsesis," she said proudly and coquettishly in her pretty Spanish accent, "I recently graduated from a special course and was hired as an accountant in Sears. I make twelve dollars an hour, have full benefits, and—guess what?—this month is the last month I will be using a welfare card. Starting next month I am going to have private insurance, and you are going to get cash from me."

I did not quite understand what she meant by the word "cash"— surely, the insurance company was going to pay the bills—but she pronounced the word "cash" with real gusto—indeed, she seemed to be really enjoying the thought of her coming financial independence. A wage of twelve dollars per hour meant a new life for Alfonsa.

I congratulated Alfonsa on her progress and cautiously reminded her about our deal. "I have been faithful to our deal," she answered. "I do not use drugs any longer. I started using drugs when I was eighteen; I got involved with them it because my brothers, my sisters, and my husband all used to deal drugs. Shortly after I delivered my twins—it was about the time when you and I met—my husband and I, together with our kids, moved to a separate household. Frankly speaking, though I had at that time made the decision not to use drugs any longer, I was pressured by my husband to continue taking drugs with him: he insisted that if I really loved him, I would keep him company in this. After about a month, however, I realized that using drugs made me feel very guilty and sick. I also suddenly understood that the more I used drugs, the more I needed them. The moment came when I could not cope any longer. I did not want to become a vegetable; not one, but three children now needed my care. My little daughters were a month old when my best friend that I had practically grown up with died from an overdose of cocaine. I remember sitting at her wake and thinking about my life—past, present, and future. It was a turning point for me: I reached my final decision not to have anything more to do with drugs.

"Who could be a mother to my children if I dropped dead?" Mrs. Cervantes asked rhetorically, and, not waiting for my response, she answered herself: "Nobody can replace a mother. That was my decision, and I have stood by it until this very day.

"My husband was unhappy that I would not keep him company, but I told him that either we lived together and took care of our children, or we parted. There was no other way.

"Now I make twelve dollars an hour, I am an independent woman, my children are healthy and well. My husband chose to stay with me and to quit drugs, though he still has not stopped completely.

"I am glad it's all behind me. Only two years ago I thought that my life was over. All I cared about was drugs, drugs, drugs. I am grateful to my parents that they did not throw us out of their house and, instead, helped me to take care of my children."

I told Alfonsa that I was more than glad to hear about her achievements.

"Doctor," she told me cheerfully, "I want to give you something that my son brought home from school. I know you will appreciate it and I would like you to keep it, please."

I took the piece of paper Alfonsa handed me. In large letters, written in red marker in a childish hand, it said only one sentence: "Say 'No' to Drugs." I hung this sign in the most visible spot in my office.

AN OLD LEATHER PURSE

I COULD hardly even remember the name of eight-year-old Amado Knudson when his mother called my office in the evening, imploring me to come to the emergency room in order to "take care" of her son, who, as far as I could understand from her excited explanation, had been brought to the hospital for a drug overdose.

Amado, who had not visited my office for more than three years, was now of the age where most children begin seeing a doctor in a practice for adults.   Though I could not remember Amado's face, I quickly recollected Alma Knudson from when she had brought her son to my office.   Alma was a polite and warm individual.

I arrived in the emergency room a short time later.   Alma Knudson was a single mother, and Amado was her only son.   She met me with a weak, unhappy smile on her face.   She was casually dressed and still carried a big, old leather purse, which I had never seen her without for as long as I had known her.   She carried this bag either by its wide strap or by just pressing it with her right lower arm.   Her face was now pale and tired.   There was no trace of makeup on it.   She paced like an animal between the room where her son lay, to the nurses' station, to the corridor, and then back to the room.   Meanwhile I was receiving a report on her son's condition from the physician on duty in the ER.

Amado had been brought in by paramedics for an overdose of some kind of illegal drugs.   Because he was not fully conscious, Amado could not remember for sure what drugs he had used, but the clinical indications pointed to PCP.

After a short report from the doctor, I went into Amado's room, accompanied by Alma and a nurse.   Amado lay on a cart, restrained, to protect him and those who were taking care of him.

I had been ready for nearly anything, but not for what I saw before me.   From Amado's clothes and his appearance I understood that he was a transvestite.   How could I hope to remember him from before, when I saw him as he was now dressed—in women's bizarre clothing and with long, permed hair done up in barrettes?   The most unnatural and aesthetically repulsive aspect of his appearance was his lips, covered with a thick layer of lipstick—by the time he had been brought to the ER, this lipstick had become so smeared that it made his mouth look like a big red hole.   The spittle drooled from this red hole as he uttered curses, profanities, and inarticulate sounds.

Amado wore a big iron cross around his neck, and his ears held long, gold-plated earrings that had what looked like satanic images on them.   Though I could not recollect what Amado used to look like, I knew for sure that he had never presented himself as a parody of a human being; he had never looked like an evil clown when he visited my office in the old days.

Amado, who was still high on drugs, did not recognize me, but when he noticed his mother, he became very agitated, until Alma removed herself from his field of vision. He was very uncooperative as I tried to examine him, struggling constantly to free himself from the restraints.

Amado had already been examined by a psychiatrist and now remained in the ER awaiting transfer to a floor where appropriate surveillance could be provided for him.

I stood next to Alma but did not want to ask her any questions. It was not a good time for her, and she was not in a position to maintain a conversation.

When it came time to transfer Amado to the psychiatric unit, he needed to be shifted from one gurney to another. The release of the restraints awakened and agitated him. Four strong people were required to move him. Using some of the filthiest profanity I had ever heard, Amado demanded to be released from the hospital. He became more and more excited and finally managed to wrestle himself away from the people who were holding onto him. Then he sat up on the cart, staring at everyone in the room, looking like a repulsive character from a Fellini film, and began to scream.

While he was fighting with the people who were restraining him, he was spluttering saliva from his red mouth and spreading rouge on his cheeks as he howled, "Faggots! Queers! Bitches! Dirty sh...y faggots!"

There was no doubt that in all his pitiful misery, in his need for self-assertion, Amado was looking for somebody who was "below" him. Though to me, he himself looked like an effeminate homosexual, by some uncanny logic he considered himself to be some "other" type. His type was superior to homosexuals, and he expressed his deep hatred for them.

Amado, who was under the influence of drugs, was giving me a lesson in the origin of scapegoating among people. Instead of homosexuals, he could have chosen some other targets for his boiling anger. Whomever he chose to blame—African Americans, Chinese, Cubans, Jews, Koreans, Mexicans, Wasps—they would not be him, who was the main culprit of his misery. The scapegoat, whom he could put lower than the gutter he was in, could always be conveniently found.

Forgotten by everyone, poor Mrs. Knudson stood in the corner of the room, stretching her neck toward her son like some big bird. It was obvious that this was not the first time her son had brought her to the emergency room; she stood like a statue, now pressing her purse to her chest; not a muscle moved on her face, her cheeks sagged, and the corners of her mouth drooped.

She caught my glance and moved toward me, asking me to step out into the corridor with her. "I want to show you something, Doctor," she said, holding me by the elbow. "Believe me, I hate my son for all that he is doing to himself, to his life, to me. I hope he forgives me for that. But I still do love my old Amado, my real son."

She picked up her big leather purse and opened it. There she quickly found what she was looking for—a pile of old photographs bound tightly by a rubber band.

She spread the photos on the counter in front of us and chose the ones she thought would best help me to remember Amado—Amado as he used to be, before he became addicted to chemicals.

"Now do you remember my wonderful child, Amado, for whom I would happily give my life, and what he looked like?" she asked me in a voice filled with emotion as I looked at the old pictures.

At this moment I saw something small and shining drop on one of the photographs Mrs. Knudson held in her hand. I looked at her face and realized that a tear had fallen on the most precious thing Mrs. Knudson had left—a memento of her priceless memories.

BIRTHDAY PRESENT

MISERY LIKES company: even when the partner in a conversation does not experience the same misery, people who have lived through an emotional crisis have a deep, internal need to share their worries and frustrations with another human being. All that is necessary to make people speak of their troubles is to demonstrate a genuine interest in, and attention to, what they are saying.

Seven-year-old June Brinstone had been brought in for a mild case of bronchitis. She used to be a frequent visitor to my office only three years earlier; then suddenly, for some unknown reason, she had stopped coming in. Since the last visit June had grown so much that I was unable to recognize her.

Her mother, Ms. Olivia Brinstone, who had worked for many years as an employment officer for a large corporation, accompanied her. Time had not been kind to Ms. Brinstone's appearance. Her complexion had changed from beautiful and outstanding to ordinary, she had bags under her eyes, and wrinkles had managed to make their way onto her forehead. I found myself involuntarily comparing her present appearance with the one still in my memory. Seven years ago, when she had first come to my office with her daughter, she had won the hearts of all who saw her with her beauty and grace. Looking at Olivia, I remembered a story I had been told of a saint. His disciples observed that his eyes were full of tears when he looked at a young, outstandingly beautiful woman. They asked him the reason for such a reaction, and he answered that he could not believe that such an example of beauty and of God's perfection could be subject to age and illness like any other mortal being.

I expressed my satisfaction to Olivia on seeing her and June again after such a long period of time and inquired whether there had been any special reason for June not coming to the office for all this time.

"Since we last saw you, Doctor, many things have happened. The majority of them were bad, but there were some good as well," Ms. Brinstone answered.

"I know that I look awful," she continued, and the shadow of a smile turned up the corner of her lips. "Don't deny it—as a woman, I could read it in your eyes when I came into the room, but I am glad just to have June around me and simply to be alive."

"Please, tell me what happened," I asked, looking into her dark, intense eyes.

"Oh, Doctor, you've probably heard stories like mine many times," Olivia answered.

"No, your story is the only one in the whole world that matters right now. Just tell me."

"Actually there is not much to say," Olivia said in a soft voice. "The last four years of my life were stolen away, and the thief was me—myself. I stopped doing drugs only five months ago. My life on drugs was one long, monotonous, gray day: high, low, high, low, and then, low, low, low."

At this moment I gave a significant glance in June's direction.

"Don't worry," Olivia said, "June knows it all already. She was there to see it all. I know this is not an excuse, but I got hooked on cocaine at the insistence of my husband. He kept telling me the same thing all the time, that if I didn't share his drug trips with him, I didn't love him. Right up to this time no one at his or my work has ever suspected us of using drugs, and he is a fireman! Gradually I got sick and tired of trying to hide my vice from everybody, including myself. But, if not for June, I might not be here now. Everything had lost any meaning to me by then, except for her. June was being taken care of by my parents; I would see her less and less frequently; the drugs froze my feelings, but the constant guilt that I was a bad mother did not go away even when I was high on drugs. This guilt gradually became more and more sharp; it was literally choking me.

"I remember my mother and father, who are not young people, begging me on their knees, yes, on their knees, to stop taking drugs, but I was as stubborn as a mule—nothing could persuade me. Five months ago our relatives called to let us know that my husband's brother who lived in California was dying of lung cancer. My husband went to see him for a week.

"In his haste he forgot to leave any drugs for me, and I did not have any idea how to get them. I gradually started to go into withdrawal.

Three days later I forgot to turn off the burner from under a boiling teakettle. June did not realize that the water in the teakettle was hot; she received second-degree burns on her right shoulder and chest. I called the paramedics; they came right away and took June to the hospital. I was sitting with June in the hospital, feeling miserable and helpless. My wonderful, good daughter was trying to bother me as little as possible. One night while I was fully conscious, I had terrible shaking in my arms and my legs. I did not want to give myself up—I needed to be close to my daughter, it was my only salvation—so I went through this horrible experience without professional help and made it, cold turkey. I prayed to God, though I don't go to church, and I promised God that if I survived I would never poison myself with drugs again.

"You don't want to hear about the hell I went through. In normal circumstances I would have needed to go to a detox center to get myself through the withdrawal period, but with June in the hospital I couldn't back off. I wouldn't blame June's doctor if he considered me a zombie. Indeed, I acted like a zombie, but I was a zombie with a goal—to become a normal, caring mother again.

"June was discharged four days later, but it took me another two or three weeks, every day of which I was afraid I was going to drop dead, to feel normal again. One day I looked in the mirror, which I had been afraid to do for years, and saw that I was still alive—shattered, beaten, deformed, but alive. I was finally in a position to give my child a normal childhood; the unrelenting iron grip of guilt started to ease its grasp from my neck. I learned that there is no greater pain than emotional pain. It would be better to be physically tortured or mutilated than to ever get on that emotional roller-coaster again.

"I then went through a divorce. Even now my husband is on drugs; he could give me up, give up our marriage, the opportunity to be with his daughter every day, but he could not give up his drugs. Many times he told me how devoted he was to our family, but he could not stop using coke and still insisted that if I really loved him, I would take coke with him. He just could not believe that I was out of that game for good.

"That's the story. I know my daughter is not that sick, but today is my birthday. If not for June, I would not be here. My love for her saved my own life. I knew that my life was worth fighting for. When I was going through my agony, I made myself a promise, that when I recovered, I would come with June to you, her pediatrician, on my birthday. For me, this is a token that I am alive again. It's my birthday present."

DEDICATED TO AMELIA

WORKING WITH people inevitable leads to stressful situations. One bright summer day the father of a patient of mine, Mr. Martin, came in during working hours to discharge himself of the tension, anger, and frustration that he accumulated somewhere other than our office.

On seeing me as I passed through the waiting room, he approached me and, in the presence of the patients, began to yell accusations at me while waving his thick thumb in front of my nose. It took some time for me to grasp what he was talking about: he was accusing me of treating his son for the wrong condition. Allegedly, I had diagnosed his child as having an ear infection when it had really been bronchitis, according to the family physician who examined the child two weeks later.

Because Mr. Martin was beyond a doubt intoxicated with drugs, alcohol, or both—I wasn't sure—my efforts to stop this barely intelligible verbal abuse were ineffective. A medical assistant who had been trying to reason with Mr. Martin before he accosted me witnessed his escalating anger and was ready to call the police. Then I noticed one of the mothers who had been sitting in the waiting room along with two of her sons; she literally jumped out of her chair to rush toward Mr. Martin.

This woman was Amelia Tyles, the mother of seven-year-old Howell and five-year-old Kevin. Amelia was thin and fragile-looking. She had black hair which she wore in a braid. Her skin was fair, but a childhood accident left a scar on her right cheek. She wore glasses with strong, thick lenses. Whenever I saw her smile, I had the feeling that her eyes radiated natural kindness.

Amelia's two children were regular visitors to our office. During these visits Amelia was helpful and unobtrusive. Her most remarkable feature was her sweet, feminine, almost singing speech, which reminded me of the speaking voice of the actress Diane Keaton. In certain situations the usually reserved Amelia had been able to take an active part in lively conversations and had demonstrated that she had a good sense of humor.

At the moment when Mr. Martin was bullying me, however, she was not at all the Amelia I knew. She reminded me of an enraged tigress pouncing in defense of her offspring. Despite her physical inadequacy, she was trying to assault Mr. Martin and was shrieking at him in a loud and angry voice, which, in a short time produced a surprising effect. Mr. Martin, who, with his bull-like, bloodshot eyes, had been boiling over with rage an instant before, suddenly became sheepishly obedient and, without saying another word, left the office in a flash. Amelia silently returned to her seat and stroked her children's heads to allay their fear.

Since a very young age I had been used to relying on my own strength when someone attacked me. This unexpected help from Amelia touched me deeply and it took me back to my very early years when my parents or my brother had come to my aid during one of my few fights.

Amelia and I became friends after this, and during her visits to the office we shared the news of our lives.

Amelia worked as a secretary at a large corporation. She was married, but I had never met her husband, Ron, who was an auto mechanic. On several occasions I inquired about him, and her answer was always that he did not come to the office because he was a busy man.

The fact that Ron did not come with his family to my office in itself proved nothing—the Tyles children were no different from any other well-adjusted children, and Amelia herself was an embodiment of self-assurance and serenity.

Three years passed. One rainy day Amelia came with her children for some simple problems. She looked unusually tired and lacked her usual vitality. I asked her the reason for the change in her appearance. With a sigh, she told me that she had recently became seriously depressed and was taking some medications that her doctor had prescribed. Though they helped her, they also decreased her energy. Though Amelia smiled an apologetic smile, she could not hide the pain in her eyes.

We met again a year later. I am not sure why Amelia was so open with me during this encounter: maybe she needed to share her problems with someone who she thought cared about her.

Though she was now taking Lithium—a strong psycholeptic medication—she still suffered from bouts of depression. During this visit I first learned some completely unexpected news—Amelia told me that she had been hospitalized recently for more than a month with a drinking problem. Nevertheless, Amelia continued with a gentle smile, her alcohol problem was in the process of being resolved. She was going to begin attending meetings at the local Alcoholics Anonymous group on a regular basis.

Though she was trying to reassure me—and herself—behind the thick lenses of her glasses I could see the tears at the corners of her eyes.

I expressed my sympathy and offered Amelia my help whenever she needed it.

Her children got older, and their visits became less frequent.

On two more occasions, as far as I could tell, Amelia's problems were lingering despite her reassurances to the contrary. It was hard to observe this kindly and pleasant woman gradually becoming a victim to her progressing alcoholism.

The last time I met Amelia was a year ago. In the middle of a busy day I was called by the receptionist to the front desk to meet "a personal visitor." Not knowing exactly who this "personal visitor" was, I came out to the reception desk and saw waiting for me a woman who appeared to be in her forties. I could read a history of long suffering on her face. Only after I looked more closely could I recognize the familiar radiant eyes behind the thick lenses and the sweet smile. Yes, it was my old friend Amelia, who alas had faded like a flower and looked ten years older than her age.

Like two old friends we embraced each other without speaking.

Time and the lifestyle that Amelia had chosen had been merciless to her. Though her figure remained good, and she still walked with her chin as high as she had nine years earlier, the freshness and charm of youth were gone from her face forever. Her appearance betrayed a life lived without enough sunshine, fresh air, or joy but, instead, filled with guilt and unhappiness.

Though the office was full of patients, I held my phone calls and apologized to the patients who were waiting for me for the short delay. I took Amelia by the arm, and we went to my office.

Looking straight into my eyes, still speaking in the lovely voice that the years had not changed, Amelia apologized that she had not appeared for so long a time—her children had grown up.

"I came to get some health information for Howell's school records and thought I should say hello to you," Amelia said in conclusion.

I thanked her and asked how she was doing.

"Fine, fine, no problems," Amelia answered quickly.

"How is your depression?"

"It is still with me. I keep taking pills to control it. They are helping."

"And what about the alcohol? I thought about you often and wanted to believe that you were no longer struggling with this problem."

Amelia paused and closed her tired eyes. I saw that she had long, beautiful eyelashes, that I had never noticed before. She sighed and answered with a short "No." and then, seeing my questioning look, continued, "I still struggle with it. But I am going to win."

"How are your husband and kids?"

"Ron and I were divorced a year ago. The kids are big now. They are really fine. You would not recognize them," Amelia said with a lovely smile, and then added quickly in a voice that suddenly became very low, "I see them very frequently." A spasm of pain distorted her face, but the smile quickly reappeared.

"I don't understand. You mean they are not with you, Amelia?" I asked gently.

"No, they are not with me. They are with Ron."

I tried in vain to find the appropriate words for this woman whose heart, as I well knew, was filled with love and tenderness. I saw a deep human tragedy before me. I could touch and talk with Amelia, but I could not reach into her very self to help her. We were close, but we were separated by an eternity. I knew that Amelia's own inability to control her weakness for alcohol had brought such pain and suffering to her children, to her ex-husband, and to herself—yes, it was her own fault. But I could not remain indifferent to the self-destruction of a person with a warm and tender heart whom I had once known so well and who had once tried to defend me. Hopefully, the other members of her family had a chance for healthy survival, but Amelia was losing hers.

I could not say a word and, with pain in my heart, I looked at Amelia, whom I could not help.

Bright red spots, caused by her nervous embarrassment, began to appear and then covered Amelia's prematurely aged face. On seeing her misery, I stretched my hand out to her. Amelia frantically grasped it; her chin started to quiver. Though I had remained silent, Amelia assumed something that I had never said and never meant to imply with my silence. In an agitated, choked, hysterical voice—the one that I heard nine years earlier when she was protecting me from an unruly patient—she shrieked, "The children are with Ron, not with me, only because they, they themselves, told me that it was better for them that way! Otherwise they would be with me. Do you believe me? Please, please, believe me, Dr. Tsesis!"

"Yes, I believe you, Amelia. I do believe you."

Though I have not seen Amelia since her unexpected visit, each time I am called to the front desk for "a personal visitor," I expect to see Amelia, the one who could defend me from a hoodlum but could not protect herself from herself. When she comes, I hope that she will give me one of her unforgettable smiles and, in her sweet voice, tell me good news about herself and her family. She will be back.

11

OBVIOUS DIAGNOSES, OBVIOUS FACTS

O ne of the exciting things about a career in pediatrics is the opportunity to establish a correct diagnosis using only minimal means—just logical thinking. One can sometimes resolve a problem that moments earlier had produced great anxiety and tension in the patient's family and can also save them time and money. It is really rewarding to see the relief in the faces of parents to whom a child's condition seemed incomprehensible only a moment earlier. They are often surprised that they were unable to see the obvious reason for the problem themselves.

HI-C DRINK

I REMEMBER an overweight eight-year-old girl who came to my office with complaints of persisting "chest pain" located behind the breastbone. After taking a careful history, I established that the reason for this pain was the liberal use of vinegar in her diet. To facilitate her weight loss, she had been eating a lot of salads, and her mother had been generously seasoning them with vinegar. As a result, large quantities of vinegar eventually produced enough irritation of her esophagus to radiate pain in correspondent part of her body—her breastbone. A full recovery followed when, on my advice, the amount of the vinegar in the patient's diet was sharply reduced.

I recalled this case when, seven years later, Margaret O'Malley brought her eleven-year-old daughter, Darlene, into my office.

Darlene was complaining of chest pain, a condition she had suffered from for at least one month. I had not seen Darlene in three years, and in that time she had been transformed from an ordinary youngster into a beautiful young lady whose appearance radiated tenderness and innocence.

After taking a history, I began a physical examination and, to my surprise, realized that the pain that she called "chest pain" was actually localized in the area of the stomach, below the rib margin and in the area of the epigastrium. There were no other findings during the physical examination.

The main way to discover the cause of abdominal pain is usually a thorough history from the patient. With this in mind, I resumed my questioning. Unfortunately, both Darlene and Margaret were not very forthcoming. Margaret belonged to the sizable group of people who think that a physician has the gift of extrasensory perception and can ascertain facts just by peering into a patient's face.

A routine blood test and other auxiliary attempts to establish a diagnosis did not bring me any closer to a solution. Not having a better explanation, I muttered that Darlene probably had a "sensitive stomach," which was reacting to something in her diet. This led us to an extensive analysis of Darlene's diet but did not help illuminate the problem.

Exhausted, I was ready to give up, when Margaret changed the subject and innocently asked me whether I thought it was a good idea to give Darlene a flu vaccine in order to prevent her from catching "a cold" during the winter months. Before I could answer, she diligently informed me that she had already undertaken some antiflu measures on her own—during the last month, on a regular basis, she had been giving Darlene a fruit juice drink enriched with vitamin C.

The red flag went up. I startled and then assumed the pose of a tiger who was preparing for a decisive pounce. Trying to sound as much as possible like the television detective Columbo, I asked Margaret to give me the details of this antiflu initiative. Mrs. O'Malley soon gave me the main piece of evidence that confirmed my diagnosis beyond any reasonable doubt: not only was Darlene being given Hi-C to drink, but she was also receiving 1,000 milligrams of vitamin C mixed into the drink. I thought to myself that this amount of vitamin C—really, a dose such as a large-animal veterinarian might prescribe—would probably perforate my stomach after the first day.

I gave my visitors my diagnosis, "gastritis, man-made," and expressed my admiration for Darlene's cast-iron stomach. Ten days later Mrs. O'Malley called to let me know that Darlene had completely recovered from her abdominal pain and also remained free of respiratory diseases.

LOWER BACK PAIN

ANOTHER CASE that required only simple detective work to diagnose was Keith Witt's. At sixteen years of age, Keith seemed to be twice as big as me—a young giant with a body of bulging muscles. He was accompanied by his mother, Norma Witt, a plump woman in her late forties who participated in the conversation far more than Keith himself. I found Mrs. Witt to be an intelligent woman who lacked a strong sense of humor.

Keith's visit was motivated by lower back pain, which he had suffered from for the last two days. His physical examination did not elicit anything unusual; it only confirmed his complaint. At sixteen years of age this complaint is rare; therefore, believing that there must be some reason for this problem, I resumed taking the history that I had begun before the physical exam. With Keith making only minimal efforts to communicate, Mrs. Witt did most of the talking and served as a "translator" when any question was directed to Keith.

After ruling out athletic activities as a reason for his complaint, we proceeded to another possibility, his work, which I thought was a promising direction. Indeed, Keith had been working from a young age. Big and strong, he worked for the owner of a neighborhood grocery store, handling heavy boxes with juice and pop bottles. I was ready to jump on this obvious diagnosis when Norma told me that Keith had stopped working at the store two weeks earlier, after a case of Coke had fallen on his leg; the resulting injury had prevented him from working since. After several more questions Keith's job was fully exonerated as the cause for his lower back pain.

We moved to the next possible cause, and I inquired about the mattress Keith slept on. Again, I was initially encouraged upon hearing that Keith slept on a mattress that was very soft and sagged under his heavy weight. Here, Norma took the opportunity to ask whether she could make the mattress firmer by placing a wide board between the mattress and the box spring. I tried to figure out how a board between the soft mattress and the box spring could possibly help but came to nothing meaningful. When I finally expressed reserved skepticism about this endeavor, Norma first agreed with me eagerly and then, like a broken record, returned to the same idea in telling me that many people from her workplace who had suffered from lower back pain had benefited from this procedure.

As Mrs. Witt shared more of her inexhaustible knowledge of popular laymen's myths and old wives' tales, I came to the realization that the "mattress theory" did not really explain Keith's lower back pain, as he had been sleeping on the same mattress for the last six years.

While I was pondering this problem, Norma, seeing my deep mental concentration, turned to Keith and, as if she had never stopped talking to him to speak with me, introduced an unexpected twist into the discussion. "Keith, maybe you got your pain on the Saturday you were working in the backyard?" To this query I heard a strong and unexpected "yes" from Keith, whose conversational skills were about as poor as he was good in helping his parents around the house.

Following this new lead, I was told that two days before, Keith had spent the entire day in his parent's backyard carrying heavy loads of topsoil back and forth in a large wheelbarrow. The puzzle was solved, and I enthusiastically confirmed Norma's guess, but she hesitated to share my professional excitement. This solution looked too simple for her.

I will never be able to figure out why some people not only refuse to accept obvious explanations but are even made uncomfortable by them.

A LUMPY PELVIC BONE

TWELVE-YEAR-OLD Cornelius Ausubel was accompanied to my office by his mother. He had a look of deep suffering written on his healthy young face. Before I could get seated at my desk, Cornelius declared in a solemn voice filled with martyrdom, "Doctor, I have a big lump on my side, and it hurts."

I looked in the direction Cornelius was pointing, and from the distance that separated us, it indeed appeared that there was a big, tumorlike formation protruding from his right side. "A tumor at this age?" The question flashed through my mind like lightning.

With my hands nearly shaking with nervous tension, I began to palpate the formation, only to discover that the "tumor" was the normal anatomical formation of the pelvic bones—the protruding ridge of its anterior and upper portion—which was sticking out from his right side just as it was appropriately designed by nature.

Both Cornelius and his mother, Mayra, accepted the good news of the absence of a tumor with reserved optimism; they were waiting for an explanation for the tenderness in this "normal anatomical formation."

I checked the sore area in a meticulous manner but could not find anything unusual. There should have been a simple explanation; Cornelius, however, was in no position to help me—he was still seeing himself as a patient in a cancer ward, and this vision was paralyzing his mind. After hearing his constant "no" to all my questions, I felt that I needed to use a special technique, one that is usually successful in making a patient's head work more actively.

With body language and gestures I let Mayra know that what I was going to say to Cornelius should not be taken too literally. In a solemn voice I intoned, "Well, then, Cornelius, you will probably need to have a lot of tests, and you and your mother will be spending a lot of time running from specialist to specialist. Some of the procedures will be quite uncomfortable and may be painful."

Even before I was through with my tirade, I could sense that the neurons in Cornelius's head had started to click in a powerful and active manner. In another moment he remembered the most obvious reason for the soreness in his pelvic bone. As it turned out, Cornelius and his younger brother shared a bunk bed. The bunk bed had a ladder, and Cornelius hit himself against it each time he passed it to get to his dresser. As Cornelius told me this, he was trying to put a little blame on his mother, as he clearly felt she was the one accountable for the inconvenient placement of furniture in his bedroom. A silent scene followed. My visitors soon left with a prescription for aspirin.

ABSOLUT

SOMETIMES IT is not the logical identification of a medical condition, but instead an obvious fact of life, to which a parent might be blind.

I first met Bridget Mellman in the emergency room of the local hospital when she was only one and a half years old. Her parents, Tina and Joel, both around twenty five years of age, appeared to be worried and alarmed by their daughter's illness. Bridget was the second child in the family. Their son Devin was three years old at this time; he had never been seriously sick.

Bridget had a severe form of bronchiolitis, a condition usually produced by a respiratory syncytial virus, a type of a virus that frequently leads to different degrees of respiratory distress in young children. Bridget was hospitalized and rapidly improved after three days of intensive treatment. She was discharged in good condition, and had been a frequent visitor to my office since then. After two more episodes of bronchiolitis, she began to show symptoms of bronchial asthma. During the cold months, I sometimes saw her two or three times a week. Frequently, Tina and Joel—perfect parents who meticulously followed my orders and provided excellent care for their daughter—would come in with Bridget, who would be wheezing, choking, coughing, and crying. Tina, who had spent a sleepless night caring for Bridget, would have red eyes, and her swollen face would have an unhealthy, yellowish coloring. Frequently, at these times, she would be tired, worried, and edgy, but knowing her well, I knew that this was not caused by any personal conflict but only by Bridget's poor condition.

For Bridget, who was growing up, time was the best healer. Phone calls from Tina gradually became less frequent and less urgent after Bridget turned three. Two more children were born to the Mellman family: a son, Arnold, and then a daughter Rita. Fortunately, they, as their brother, Devin, were almost never sick. I saw Bridget in my office both when she accompanied her siblings for their exams and during her own regular checkups.

When Bridget was six, she came to my office for a minor skin problem. She was accompanied by her mother, sister, and the younger brother. Her father, who owned a small carpet cleaning business, did not come with the family, as he usually did when he was not too busy at his work. Bridget behaved like an old customer, expecting maximum attention, which she definitely got. Her mother looked healthy, content, and at least ten years younger than she had during the time of Bridget's illness. Tina had the appearance of a person who knew that she was doing something meaningful and important with her life, which, for her, was the rearing of her four children. She had an attractive appearance on this day, dressed in a pretty, neat, blue T-shirt and designer jeans that enhanced her graceful, slim body. Her hair was done in good taste.

Bridget sat on the exam table throwing me nervous and distrustful looks—she was expecting some shots, though I had emphatically assured her more than once that we were saying "no" to "dirty tricks" of the medical trade. At least for this visit. Her brother and sister were involved in a lively "conversation" in the exam room as well.

Bridget's skin problem turned out to be quite simple and soon the Mellmans were ready to depart. While I was explaining to Tina how to use the prescribed medication, I thought to myself how young and pretty she looked that day, but something in her outfit I was unable to name annoyed me. To figure out what it might be, I scanned Tina's attire until the culprit was found, and thus there was a pause in the conversation.

"Is something wrong?" Tina asked.

In a small private practice, where the family has known their physician for many years, conditions are favorable for frank and open discussion, which may not be possible even among members of the family. If not for the many years I had treated Tina's family, which resulted in a relation of trust, I would not have elaborated on the reason for my pause, but with Tina I could answer sincerely.

"Well, Tina, let me ask you. Do you support alcohol abuse and the glamorization of alcohol usage?" I answered her with a question.

"No. Why?" Tina replied promptly, waiting impatiently for an explanation.

"Would you agree to promote the use of alcohol for money or on a voluntary basis?" I asked her.

"Of course not! Tell me, why are you are asking these questions?"

"I remember how, a while back, you came in wearing a button that read, 'Say No to Drugs'; now I see that you are promoting the opposite side of the issue." I pointed to an elegant, artistic logo in the upper right corner on her T-shirt:

Be Resolute
Drink
ABSOLUT

"I like the T-shirt, but not the message," I said.

"I never thought about the message," Tina answered simply and sincerely, "Why, do you think it might be harmful?"

"When you were wearing the 'Say No to Drugs' pin, you were expecting a positive effect from that message. Otherwise, why wear it? By the same token, don't you think that the 'Absolut' sign is an endorsement of alcohol?"

For me, what I was saying to Tina was so obvious that I expected her to interrupt me with an impatient "I know," but, instead, she was all attention.

Because of her interest, I continued. "I know the reality, Tina. I see alcohol promoting signs constantly on shirts, jackets, pants, sweaters, which adults and older children wear. I am sure they are blind to the fact that they are a part of a big propaganda machine. I am not in a position to tell them my ideas on this matter, but with you, a dedicated mother and a friend of mine, I feel I should share this opinion. We live in a time of rapid, radical changes in our society, when the values once so familiar to us all are now frequently confused and perverted. No one can guarantee that your children will never experiment with alcohol at some point. If, God forbid, any of them choose to abuse alcohol, as so many teenagers, unfortunately, do, you want, for the sake of your own conscience, to be able to say that was not a value that you had supported or promoted."

I stopped, feeling that what I was saying required no additional explanation. I waited for Tina's reaction.

"Someone gave me this shirt as a present. I never drink alcohol more than socially. I never paid attention to the logo on the shirt," she said with a sparkle in her eyes.

I decided that we were going nowhere: as has happened on some other occasions, my intentions had been misunderstood, and I decided to close the subject and said good-bye.

Unexpectedly, Tina understood my reaction. The tone of her voice was pressing. "Please, understand me properly," she said. "I really never put these things together. Now it is obvious to me." She paused and then continued. "I am really grateful to you for your time and your desire to tell me this. You did not waste your time on this with me. You are right. Absolutely."

12

EXPELLING THE PROBLEM

Vomiting—one of the symptoms that pediatricians encounter most frequently in their day-to-day practice—is caused by many various illnesses and frequently presents a diagnostic challenge to the pediatrician. The most frequent condition that is accompanied by vomiting is commonly known as intestinal flu.

"Intestinal flu," which occurs all year round but is most common during the winter months, created for us in the office a continual budget drain in the form of having to replace the carpeting frequently—until I had an excellent idea. I eradicated this problem by placing plastic business chair mats in all the potential "danger zones" of the office.

In the majority of cases the discussion of vomiting is not usually a subject for smiles—especially when it is the bothersome condition that is known as psychogenic vomiting, that is, vomiting caused by emotional conflicts.

Parental divorce is nowadays a frequent cause of mental tension for children. Though the degree of damage that this now regular social occurrence has on a child's psyche varies case to case, divorce always has a deep influence on the innocent parties—the children, whose main attitude to the world of adults is trust. Divorce, where the most predictable people a child knows split the child's world apart, presents an undisputed and serious break in this trust.

If divorce were a disease, its stages could be identified as acute and chronic. The most traumatic stage, the acute, takes place at the time of the divorce; the chronic stage continues for the rest of a child's life.

Although many parents try to help their children get through both stages with the least possible emotional shock, frequently, parents can be so preoccupied with their own emotional wounds that they sometimes lose sight of their children's pain. Indeed, in some cases they make the situation the child is in much worse than it needs to be.

Over the years I have discovered for myself that vomiting may frequently serve as one of the objective signs of a child's psychological distress. Psychoanalysts give numerous theories for this symptom; trying to simplify things for my own understanding of this clinical sign, I explain it as a subconscious desire of the child to expel the problem out of sight, out of mind.

CONFIRMED DIAGNOSIS

I REMEMBER when Emily Botkin and her husband, Donald, stood together to try to save the life of their middle child, their son Stephen. Stephen was born with a severe abnormality of vertebrae and spinal cord. I had just joined the practice of my, now former, partner when Stephen was born. The Botkins had known my predecessor for six years and thus preferred to see him, but when he retired, they became my patients. Stephen was around three years old at that time.

The first time Stephen was operated on, the results were good, but about three years later he again began to exhibit the symptoms of cardiac insufficiency. He was then admitted to Children's Memorial Hospital for a possible surgical intervention because his condition was worsening.

The Botkins were a lower middle-class family. Donald Botkin was a hardworking roofer and his wife, Emily, was a busy housewife.

I was really impressed with their family unity, which was especially apparent during the time when the family was fighting for Stephen's life. During this period Donald called me twice a day, sometimes more often than that, to inform me of Stephen's progress. He even called me on the day when little Stephen died during his complicated surgery. This was the last time I ever heard from Donald.

Two months later I received a formal letter from Emily requesting that I transfer the children's records to another pediatrician. The family had moved to a far northern suburb twenty miles from my office. Before signing the records, I called the old Botkin residence, and Emily's mother answered. She told me, to my complete surprise, that not only had Emily moved but she had also filed for a divorce from Donald. I left a message for Emily but never got a call back from her.

Nearly three years later, she came into my office with her two children from her marriage to Donald and with a nine-year-old boy whom I had never met before. Emily told me that she had remarried and that Simon was her stepson. Though thin and tired-looking, Emily also seemed content and satisfied. The suffering expression of old had disappeared, attesting to the fact that she had achieved peace of mind since our last meeting.

The reason for this visit was Simon's persistent vomiting. I could not establish the cause for his symptoms and asked Emily to bring Simon back in ten days. They did not, however, return for this follow-up visit.

Out of the blue, Emily came back to my office some five years later with one of her sons and Simon. Both children had a mild case of chickenpox. Emily looked even more relaxed and at peace with herself; her second marriage was apparently working out well for her. We behaved as if we had seen each other only a few days before. Looking through Simon's chart, I recalled how five years before, I had been trying unsuccessfully to establish the reason for his vomiting. The cause was still a puzzle to me. I could not remember the details of the visit, but a note in the chart told me that my provisional diagnosis had been psychogenic vomiting.

"Do you remember, Mrs. Wolf (this was now Emily's last name), how Simon was suffering from unexplained vomiting when I examined him the last time? I suppose something must have prevented you from bringing him in for the follow-up visit?"

Emily told me that she had failed to come into the office because during that time her mother had been very ill and had died shortly thereafter. She was thus unable to keep the appointment.

"Five years have passed since that visit, but I am still not sure I was on the right track then. Was I correct when I told you that his vomiting was of a psychogenic nature?"

In her characteristic, unemotional monotone, Emily answered, "Yeah. You were right. He was vomiting because he was listening to all those arguments between my present husband and his ex-wife,

Simon's mother. Even though they were divorced, they were still settling different issues in Simon's presence and were arguing like crazy. After you said that the vomiting might be caused by all of this stuff, they kept Simon out of their arguments, and he eventually stopped vomiting."

SETTLING FOR THE MINIMUM

I OBSERVED another case of psychogenic vomiting, which resembled Simon's case, with a member of the Rafael family. The family consisted of the parents, Cecilia and Bruno, both in their late thirties, and three children, of whom Poppy, the heroine of this episode, was the youngest. Seven-year-old Poppy was a smart, nice looking, energetic child who was never seriously ill.

Cecilia, though weak in the sense-of-humor department, had a passionate Mediterranean temper but was usually friendly and cooperative with me. One day she brought her daughter for one complaint only—she had been vomiting at least three to four times a day for the last two weeks. Cecilia was very worried, especially as it seemed to her that Poppy was losing weight.

Poppy did not react much during her mother's narrative. She was sitting on the examining table and seemed to be absorbed in her thoughts while she vigorously chewed gum and energetically jiggled her legs.

Unable to find a specific reason for her vomiting, I ordered a basic laboratory workup, gave several recommendations, and said that I needed to see Poppy again in three to four days.

Four days later, Cecilia and Poppy came in again and, to my grave disappointment, I learned that her vomiting had become even worse. The results of the laboratory tests were all normal, and I did not know what to tell Cecilia about the next course of action. But, even before I began to speak, Cecilia took the matter into her own hands. With her typical intensity, she told me that she might have a good explanation of what was causing Poppy's problem. It was obvious to me that she had suspected this reason from the beginning but had decided to let me rule out other possible medical problems first and then let me know about what she considered the real cause of the problem.

After this statement, she asked Poppy to go to the waiting room and watch television. When Poppy closed the door behind her Cecilia immediately began. "It's all because of this woman that she vomits—I thought it was so, but now I am convinced!"

"Woman? You didn't mention anything about a woman. Aren't you happily married?" I asked.

"Happily married? I wish! That's all in the past. Bruno found another woman, fifteen years younger than me, no less. It has gone on for about a year. We are in the final stages of a divorce. Anyway, Poppy and the other children have thought all along that their father would change his mind about the divorce, but about a month ago he told them they should forget about that. Poppy's vomiting started then. At the time I thought it was a coincidence, but the more I think of it now, the more convinced I am that the events are related. Especially as my husband seldom sees the children, and when they do go to his new apartment, he always has this young woman around."

"Why didn't you tell me about this before! We would not have done all these tests."

Cecilia did not answer. She just spread her hands in a helpless gesture.

We decided I should talk with Bruno to try to help Poppy, and I asked Cecilia to have him come into the office.

Two days later, Bruno, Cecilia, and Poppy were sitting with me in my office. Once again I examined Poppy and again I could find no physical cause for her complaint. Her vomiting persisted.

At my request, Poppy and her mother left the room. I had never met Bruno before. He was a tall man with dark, shiny hair. He was no longer young-looking—there were bags under his eyes, he was obese, and his chubby cheeks showed their tendency to sag.

Bruno was working as a clerk at the local Immigration and Naturalization office. Whether his self-important attitude was related to his profession or to his belief that he was a young, irresistible catch, I couldn't say; his attitude, however, was definitely that of a pubescent peacock who thought himself the center of the universe. Nonetheless, I strongly felt that if Bruno could not imagine the internal torment his child was going through, he was, at least, impressed with, and upset by, Poppy's constant vomiting.

Bruno sat across from me, solemn and silent, staring into space. I explained as well as I could what I thought about the cause of his daughter's condition and asked Bruno whether he thought this could be so.

"It might be, Doc. Whatever you say," answered Bruno in a telegraphic fashion.

I repeated my supposition and then told Bruno that I thought more frequent contact with his children, especially with Poppy, and, if possible, without his girlfriend, might be of real help to them.

"Well," reacted Bruno, "to tell you the truth, Doc, I'm a very busy man. But, even though I don't believe in all this psychological crap too much, I guess I might give it a shot. At least for a while."

It was hard for me to imagine that even with his haughty attitude, Bruno, a man with a presumably normal psyche, would not be affected by the recent dramatic events in his life as were the other members of the family; I assumed that he, like anyone, might need some support. "How are *you* taking the changes. How are *you* doing?" I asked him. His answer showed how naive I can be sometimes.

"Me?" Bruno answered with a reserved but proud smile on his large face. He cleared his throat to produce the maximal effect. "Ok, Doc. I'm doing perfect. I don't know whether Poppy told you, but I was just promoted to the position of an assistant to a supervisor. I have two people and one part-timer work under me now."

Two weeks later Cecilia told me that Poppy was cured. As has happened in similar situations I have seen, Poppy had settled for the minimum for her recovery. All that she needed was to keep some of her seven-year-old human dignity intact, to know that she was not losing her father forever, and to see her father without the offending presence of the young woman who had stolen him away. A modest enough desire for a young human soul, no? Bruno had been "kind" enough to follow my advice and had been seeing his children more frequently, without his girlfriend.

My, wasn't that generous?

A SLEEPOVER

WHILE WORKING with many different people, I have had the opportunity to observe their best and worst qualities. It seems to me that some people carry in their chests not a human heart, but a piece of stone.

I remember I once shared with the mother of one of my patients how stunned I was by a girl who had come to my office earlier in the day for a sore throat; this child had pierced her own tongue with an earring. This parent, not a highly educated woman, expressed my own feelings with her comment, "How will they care about others if they hate themselves?"

By the same token, observing some parents (fortunately, these parents are a small minority), I realize that society cannot expect too much from these parents in being responsible citizens as they do not even care for their own children.

One such parent was Donovan Kern, who came into my office with his twelve-year-old daughter, April. Like the other patients in this chapter, April was suffering from persistent vomiting.

April was not a regular patient of mine. She had been referred to my office by the emergency room of a local hospital where, two days before, she had been treated because of vomiting that had been ongoing for two days. The perplexed physician had ordered many tests, including a computerized tomography scan and an upper gastrointestinal tract X ray. The results of these tests all came back normal, and the patient was discharged from the ER with a generic diagnosis of gastritis and nearly $1,000 in medical bills.

After taking a detailed history and meticulously examining April, I could find no reason for her only, but expensive, symptom. Neither April nor her father was very cooperative. Mr. Kern was more or less obediently answering my questions while volunteering no information, and his daughter seemed lost in her own deep thoughts and answered my questions with no enthusiasm. Finally, discouraged by their uncooperative attitudes, I told Mr. Kern that I was inclined to think that April's condition was psychosomatic in nature. I advised him that his daughter should avoid stressful situations and should temporarily try to follow a diet free of heavily spiced foods and coffee. We agreed that I would reevaluate April in a week.

Though I never saw April again, I did discover the real reason for her illness. April's life was literally making her sick to her stomach.

Three to four hours after April left my office, I received an urgent call from her mother, Jenny Kern.

After introducing herself, she immediately got to the point. What she had to tell me was hard to imagine. Jenny and Donovan had been divorced for two years. April and her eleven-year-old brother, Ed, lived with their mother. Under the terms of the custody agreement, however, their father had the right to visitation on the weekends.

During the children's last visit with their father they had gone to a movie and then to a favorite restaurant, where their father's young girlfriend joined them.

From the restaurant all four of them went to Donovan's apartment, and at eleven o'clock everyone went to bed. For the first time in her life April was put in the same bed with her younger brother. Both children protested, but with an innocent smile their father told them that there were, unfortunately, no other beds available.

April and her brother finally fell asleep, turning their backs to each other. Soon they were awakened by strange sounds coming through the wall separating them from the bedroom where their father and his girlfriend were. Ed, who woke first, shook April's shoulder to waken her. He was frightened by the sounds of moaning and sighing, sounds that he had never heard before. He also heard the rhythmic squeaking of the bed on the other side of the wall.

April, when she woke up, understood it all but did not want to share her knowledge with her brother. She lay in bed, holding onto Ed tightly, unable to speak until the last screams sounded from the other side of the wall.

On the next day April developed the vomiting problem.

It was hard to believe such a bizarre story. Was it possible that an educated, civilized man, a father, could be so cruel to his own children? I told Mrs. Kern that the law obliged me to report a case such as this to the Department of Children and Family Services, but she told me that she had already contacted them. Nevertheless, I placed a call to DCFS and confirmed that this case was under investigation.

Soon after, Mrs. Kern and her children moved to a far northern suburb with her mother. My office was too far away, and so she took April to a pediatrician near her home with whom I communicated by phone. The intractable vomiting from which April had suffered disappeared as soon as they moved.

I received a couple of calls from DCFS, as the agency was interested in my opinion regarding this case. Eventually a decision was made by the court to deprive the father of his visitation rights. I hope that he repented and was later able to see his children again. The memory of their father's sinful behavior, however, may stay with his children forever, reminding them that sometimes the person they trusted most might betray them, all the while wearing a smile on his face.

SECRET WEAPON

THIS STORY does not feature psychosomatic vomiting, I include it as a story that presents vomiting in an unusual light. Though vomiting is not an aesthetically pleasing act of human physiology, I remember an episode that became the subject of humorous reminiscence between the Kepler family and me.

Eleven-month-old Allen Kepler had been brought to my office for a cough and congestion. In the process of giving him a physical examination, I needed to check his throat. Allen was a stubborn baby and refused the throat exam with tightly clenched teeth. It became necessary to enlist the help of both his mother and his grandmother to restrain him.

While I tried to unlock Allen's tightly compressed teeth, I noticed something unusual. Allen was looking straight at me, shifting his gaze from one part of my face to another; he reminded me of a moving radar antenna and gave me the impossible idea that he was aiming at my face. But what weapon could this innocent and restrained child have at his disposal? In another second I learned an important professional lesson—just as I had nearly unclenched his teeth, Allen produced a loud burp, which was followed by a thick stream of the entire contents of his stomach, aimed straight at my puzzled face. I was lucky, he missed by only a fraction of an inch, with his unusual means of getting even with a pediatrician.

13

FUN WITH PEDIATRICS

For someone who is not familiar with pediatric medicine, the work of the pediatrician, working amid the incessant cries of children, might seem very stressful. Actually, the stressful part of a pediatrician's job is not crying children; like many other things in life one gets used to this. The really stressful aspect of pediatrics is high-risk cases, for example, when a child is suffering from dehydration, a persistently high fever, a severe case of croup, or an acute bronchial asthma attack. But when no patients are seriously sick, and the office is not busy with the school physical season or with the victims of a current epidemic, then the pediatrician has an opportunity not only to relax but even to have fun with the job. As a matter of fact, more pediatricians than physicians of any other specialties are intentionally limiting their workload in order to have an opportunity to communicate more with their patients. Those physicians who cannot afford to cut their workload because of financial or other considerations are still able to have some share of the delight in working with young children and, yes, with their parents, as well.

Unfortunately, the progressive bureaucratization of medicine introduced an avalanche of unnecessary paperwork, which puts an invisible barrier between the patient and physician; this is especially the case for a physician who works as an independent practitioner. This trend might gradually end a wonderful phenomenon of Western medicine—private medical offices, where conditions are most conducive to forming a good rapport between patient and physician. For the near future, private medical offices will survive, but if the pressure from the bureaucrats continues to increase, fewer and fewer physicians will be able to maintain their independent status. They will,

instead, join large group practices where they will have less opportunity to develop their individual style of medical practice.

But until this undesirable event fully engulfs the practice of pediatrics, this field of medicine remains a world of challenge and fun.
Like any other pediatrician who has spent several years in active practice, I have some stories to tell.

WAITING FOR MRS. TODAUT

ON A balmy day in July during my regular office hours, one of
the office medical assistants told me that fourteen-year-old Eduardo
Todaut had arrived. He had been suffering from warts on his palm
for a couple of months, and I had been treating them with a strong
acid solution. This was the third treatment session for Eduardo's
warts, and, so far, the warts were responding to the treatment.

Destroying warts is a procedure I like; unlike many of the conditions that I treat as a general pediatrician, the results of this surgical
treatment can be seen immediately, giving me a pleasant feeling of
professional achievement.

After I greeted both Eduardo and his mother, I examined the warts
and, to my satisfaction, found that they were disappearing. I enthusiastically shared this information with both Eduardo and his mother
as I started to prepare another application of the acid. Eduardo then
pointed out a lesion on his other hand. He injured this hand during
his wrestling class. The lesion was bleeding.

Eduardo and his mother thought that this was another wart, but
after I had examined the lesion, I had my doubts. In order to determine exactly what this lesion was, I needed to perform a biopsy. I
informed my visitors of this and began the procedure. After successfully removing a piece of tissue for the biopsy, I realized, to my cha-
grin, that the office had just run out of formalin, a tissue fixative.
Since the microscopy of the sample could not be delayed, I asked
Mrs. Todaut to take the tissue sample to a nearby hospital laboratory
right away. Otherwise the tissue, which was not preserved in fixative, might be spoiled. Mrs. Todaut and I had been friends for a long
time, and she was happy to help me. I then placed the specimen in a
sterile plastic cup, put on a reliable lid, placed it in a special enve-

lope, and handed it to Mrs. Todaut, after which my visitors left the examining room.

Ten minutes later, while passing from one examining room to another, I noticed Eduardo sitting in the waiting room. Surprised that the Todauts were still in the office, I looked for Eduardo's mother, but did not see her. Instead, sitting next to Eduardo was an older woman, who, like Eduardo, seemed to be of Italian descent. Apparently, I decided, Mrs. Todaut had gone to the hospital laboratory as she had promised, leaving her son and mother (or mother-in-law?) behind.

Why would she do that? This was a question I could not answer, but it was logical to assume that Eduardo and the woman, who was evidently his grandmother, were waiting for Mrs. Todaut to come back from the laboratory. Out of respect for grandmother's age, but especially because she was staring at me with an intent look, I, addressed her, not Eduardo, with my question about the whereabouts of Mrs. Todaut. This caused Eduardo's neighbor to look at me with even more intensity.

Answering her fixed look with similar enthusiasm and speaking in the quick rhythm of a fast-paced pediatric office, I asked her cheerfully, "Why haven't you left the office yet, Grandmother?"

To my surprise the grandmother not only did not answer my question but increased the intensity of her searching, inquisitive gaze. I repeated my question. "Why should I leave?" she eventually asked me with a provocative challenge in her voice.

"Weren't you supposed to go with your daughter to bring Eduardo's tissue specimen to Mount Zion Hospital?"

"What specimen; I do not understand you!" replied Eduardo's grandmother with indignation. Her look showed her lack of desire to continue the conversation.

I realized that our conversation, which had only just begun, had already been spoiled. I needed to get on a better footing with her and began again.

"Ok, could you just tell me where your daughter is, ma'am?" I asked her as delicately as I could.

"Why should I tell you where my daughter is?" retorted the woman, indicating with her entire appearance that she was not going to discuss family issues with me. I did not insist and addressed the question to her grandchild. Eduardo was much more cooperative.

Without delay he gave a very simple explanation of the situation. He told me that his mother had gone to the washroom and should be back any minute. I could hear that Eduardo was embarrassed for some reason; meanwhile, his grandmother continued her unrelenting, fixed stare.

Finally, having received a satisfactory explanation to my question, I did my best to finish the conversation on a peaceful and positive note. "Please, hurry up, as I want the wart specimen to be delivered to the laboratory before it gets spoiled," I said to both of them.

The grandmother maintained her incredulous look at me and then turned toward Eduardo, seeking his support in their mutual distress, and exclaimed, "What is he talking about! Warts, tissues! I am clean!" Then, turning toward me, she added with the same passion, "Just leave us alone!"

Eduardo looked still more embarrassed, and I decided that I should return to my office routine and discontinue this unexpected and unwarranted dispute.

Another forty minutes passed, and I found myself once again in the waiting room. To my great surprise, this time I saw only the grandmother, sitting by herself in my waiting room. Neither Eduardo nor his mother was around.

Trying to use the maximum amount of tact and respect with this visitor, who had spent so much time in the office, I said with a gentle smile, "Well, now they have left *you* behind and are going to pick you up on the way back from the hospital, right, Grandmother?"

Again, it did not fail—my question produced a negative reaction on the part of the woman.

"They who?" she asked me brusquely.

"Well, your daughter Mrs. Todaut and your grandson Eduardo, the one who was sitting next to you half an hour ago."

"Just for your information, I never heard those names before, and I never met this boy before. The boy just happened to be sitting next to me. And my name is Mrs. Bustle. I came to this office to see Dr. Samuel, the allergist, for my hay fever. Because of a problem I had with my ride, I came an hour earlier than my appointment was scheduled for."

Before I could open my mouth to apologize for the confusion, I heard loud laughter from my staff, who finally understood the comedy of errors that they had witnessed in the waiting room.

Mrs. Bustle accepted my apology with some hesitation. She could forgive everything except my careless remark that she should leave the office, which I had mistakenly made when I had assumed her to be a part of the Todaut family.

The last thing people want to hear is the words of rejection.

GOOD MANNERS

I STARTED to work in my present office in December 1979. At that time it was one-half of its present size and contained only one-third of the people who now work there. Nowadays, the office has six examining rooms, in which I spend many hours of my life.

In this office I have examined thousands of people and have tried, to the best of my abilities, to help them. In this office the youthful reddish-brown color of my hair gradually changed to the noble silver of the postyouth age. The office is my second home. I know each nook and cranny here. No matter how carefully my assistants clean and prepare the office, at any moment, if I wanted, I could find some kind of irregularity that would not be noticed by them.

As is my habit, I begin my morning working hours exactly at nine o'clock. In addition to my stethoscope, I am also armed with other tools of my trade—an electronic organizer, a English-Spanish translator, the electronic edition of the *Physicians' Desk Reference,* and prescription forms—all of which I carry in a little briefcase. On one June morning I entered the examining room where Mrs. Howard and her six-month-old daughter were waiting for a routine well-baby examination.

Little Lolita was cozily sucking on her "designer" pacifier, and her mother was looking at her precious daughter with admiration, while determinedly chewing gum. I was ready to start the examination when Mrs. Howard told me she was concerned that her daughter was gaining too much weight.

Maybe the problem was not with the baby, but with the scale? I looked in the direction of the baby scale and immediately noticed that something was wrong with it. It was completely out of balance, and my repeated attempts to balance it were unsuccessful. The office was busy, and other patients were waiting for me, so I could not continue my efforts to fix the scale. Through the intercom I asked the office supervisor, Galina, to come to the room. After Galina, a pleasant and softspoken woman, came in, I explained as tactfully as I could my disappointment that the scale had not been prepared before office hours began.

Galina, a thorough, hardworking person, was visibly upset about the scale malfunction, but soon, instead of looking at me as I spoke, she began stubbornly looking at the scale.

"What's the matter, Galina. Why you are looking at the scale?" I asked her, trying to get her attention.

"I am so sorry, Doctor," Galina answered in the most courteous Japanese-like manner, "but, Doctor, maybe the scale would balance better if you would kindly remove your briefcase from the top of it. Thank you very much."

I blushed.

INSEPARABLE FRIENDS

FRANNIE FELDEN was only five months old when her mother allowed her to walk in a walker. After that, little Frannie would not give up this device, which at her young age made her life more mobile and interesting.

I can never remember this child being unhappy or lacking energy. Even when she was only two months old, she was able to express her individuality and responded in the most friendly manner to those adults who were willing to talk and play with her. She started to crawl at seven months and was able to sit up without support at five months of age—two months ahead of schedule for the average child.

When Frannie was only ten months old, she was able to walk by herself, but she wanted to run and demanded to be put in the walker, which allowed her to be an active part of the world around her and gave her a feeling of freedom and joy.

During office hours Frannie's mother called me to say that her older daughter had forgotten to put the gate across the door that leads to the basement, and our poor explorer fell ten steps down the stairs while running in her walker.

I never trusted walkers and am dismayed with their potential hazard for children. A child in a walker should never be left unsupervised. Full of anxiety for Frannie's health, I ask her mother to call for paramedics right away if she had not yet done so. Instead of taking my recommendation, Mrs. Felden comforted me. "Don't worry, Doc. Frannie doesn't look bad at all. The stairs to the basement are carpeted, it is a very thick kind of carpet, and after she fell down, she clambered right back up the stairs on all fours pulling her best friend—the walker—behind her. I just want to have her checked for my own peace of mind."

A STEREO SYSTEM

NOWADAYS, PEOPLE think within electronic categories. The Smith family is a working couple with three children. One of them, Jack, is five years old. The two other children, Darrel and Carina, are ten-month-old twins. Mr. Smith usually works the night shift, and, therefore, he brings the children to the office for their examination while his wife is working during the daytime.

In the middle of the examination, Darrel and Carina were very unhappy, lying on the exam table and crying to the full capacity of their healthy lungs. From the strength of the sound waves produced by these tiny creatures, it seemed that the walls were trembling, and the ceiling was shaking.

At this noisy moment I heard Mr. Smith's fatherly voice. As he looked at his wonderful children, he said, "You see, Doc, how nice it is to have twins? Thanks to them I have a free, wireless, family stereo system that only needs to be fed regularly."

OVERPSYCHOLOGIZED

THE REASON for a smile is not always easy to explain, and sometimes it appears on the face when it should not be there at all. My excuse is that we are only humans, whether we are doctors or patients.

The mother of a two-year-old baby named Rosemary looked very concerned as she asked me why her daughter had tears in her eyes any time she peed and/or pooped.

"I would not be worried," said Rosemary's mother, "if she was sobbing or showing that she was upset in some other way. But as she sits on the potty to pee or poop, tears run down her face and all the while she might be laughing or smiling."

Having this brain-teaser before me which to the best of my knowledge had never been described in any pediatric literature, I was trying to alleviate the mother's worries with some simple reassurances, but she demanded a scientific explanation. Almost ready to capitulate I presented an overpsychologized hodgepodge of ideas taken from the theories of Freud, Piaget, and Erickson, which produced such an unexpectedly strong impression on Rosemary's mother that I began to feel I was about to burst out laughing. I started to cough, apologized, and ran out into the corridor.

ADULT TALK

FOUR-YEAR-OLD Tanya Mason likes to come into my office and does not miss an opportunity to enter into animated conversation, now and then she uses words which belong to an "adult" vocabulary. Trying to imitate her "adult" talk, with a serious face I asked Tanya whether she had given the nurse her urine specimen for the urinalysis which is required as part of the pre-school examination.

Tanya looked at me intently, trying to prepare a dignified answer. Jokingly, I asked her, "Do you know how to urinate?"

"N-n-n-o-o-o," she answered, pondering my question.

"Do you know how to pee?"

"I know how to pee, but I do not know how to urinate," Tanya replied thoughtfully.

SPEAKING OF BOYS

IN MY thirty years of working with people, I have come to the conclusion that the easiest way to deal with them is to be myself. Having made such a discovery, I do not hesitate to joke with my patients when it is relevant, and they feel free to joke with me as well.

I once asked the mother of three girls who were patients of mine why she was "prejudiced" against boys. "I have one," answered Mrs. Spencer, and a wide smile appeared on her face.

"Who is it?"

"My husband," she answered. "He is my good boy."

WHAT'S IN A NAME?

IN THESE days of brave, out-of-control experimentation with children' education, fewer and fewer children are coming to the office with books to read while they wait their turn to be examined. At most they bring a very thin book with a lot of pictures in it or try to solve one of those "challenging" find-a-word puzzles that involve circling out words from a jumble of letters. Sixteen-year-old Bunny Bregvadze's natural curiosity, however, had not been corrupted by the modern attitude to the written word; she always brought serious books to read, and, knowing my background, she enjoyed discussing with me the news of the country of my birth, the former Soviet Union.

Bunny was short and athletically built, with large, remarkable eyes and shiny, soft blond hair. Just before she came to my office she had listened to a radio program about Russia and wanted to share with me her thoughts on some of the problems in that country. Out of an hour-long program she wanted to discuss only one story, a story about her namesakes that had really cut her to the quick.

"Can you imagine," Bunny said in an excited tone. "They are in such turmoil there that somebody stole the rabbits from the Moscow zoo!"

"Poor bunnies," I echoed.

VOLUNTEERING TO BE A PATIENT

HERBERT RUTTER, a promising young man of three, was a very disciplined and orderly child. I do not ever remember this child crying; from an early age, even after injections, he would only frown momentarily and then return to his regular happy attitude.

One day he accompanied his five-year-old brother, Sheffield, to the office for a visit. Sheffield, as I had expected, turned out to be in good health. I was ready to return to my desk after completing his exam when suddenly I saw an unexpected patient. Little Herbert stripped off all of his clothes except for his briefs, and now—thin as a reed except for his protruding belly—stood silent, solemn and patient, looking at me and waiting for his turn to be examined.

Herbert was not scheduled for a visit, and he was obviously very healthy. He had evidently decided that as long as he was a legitimate patient of the office and since his older brother had taken his clothes off for an examination, it was only natural to expect that he was going to be examined as well. Seeing my smile, his father explained, "Herb likes to be examined by the doctor." Without hesitation I applied a stethoscope to Herbert's narrow chest, which promised one day to be broad and athletic.

BACK TO CLASSICAL MUSIC

FOR ME, one of the invaluable advantages of working in a private office is the opportunity to hear music of my choice. My partner and I like to listen to classical music, so we always play classical records, tapes, and CDs in the office.

Today our program consisted of Italian music. When I entered the examining room to see the next patient, I observed the everlasting power of music: two beautiful girls dressed in checkered school uniforms were frolicking and bouncing, dancing the hàbànérà from Georges Bizet's opera *Carmen*.

According to their mother, it was the first time in their lives they had heard the uplifting melody, but they obviously liked the music a lot. They were not yet old enough to think, as many children of today do, that classical music is "not cool."

GRANDMOTHER'S PRAISE

To MAKE my pediatric practice more appealing to my young patients, I introduced remote control toys and electronic gizmos, which the children love to see in the office.

Twelve-year-old Kelly Yellich, though he was not talkative or demonstrative about it, enjoyed the toy show. One day, while he watched the choo-choo train run on the track that is fixed around the perimeter of the office, I said to him, "I did it all for you, kid!" Kelly nodded his head, but, unexpectedly, his grandmother said to me as she gave a beautiful smile, "No, you did it for me, Doctor!"

THE CASE OF THE ALMOST STICKUP

ONE VERY popular item in our office is a vending machine that is placed in the waiting room area. It is loaded with small, colorful objects such as rings, toys, and stickers. These items are packaged in small capsules that are dispensed by the machine. Children love to receive a present, especially if the contents are a surprise, and few children leave the office without trying their luck on this amazingly useful tool of pediatric public relations.

The vending machine operates with special tokens that have the inscription "To a Good Child." The tokens, which are given one per visitor by a receptionist or medical assistant after the patient is treated by the pediatrician, present a strong motivating force for the patient to be more cooperative during exams and other medical procedures.

As I was completing an examination, the patient addressed words to me that might have been intimidating had they not originated from Arnold Roberson, two-and-a-half years old. While I was writing a prescription to treat his runny nose, I felt him touching my right hand with his tiny fingers, trying to get my attention.

Arnold had a demanding and uncompromising look on his face, as does a person asking for something that rightfully belongs to him.

As he stood with one hand holding up his falling jeans, he demanded, "Give me money," in a thin, childish voice which allowed for no objection on my part.

Incredulous, I asked him to repeat his statement.

"Give me your money!" reiterated my visitor with all the eloquence he had at his disposal.

My hand automatically went to the pocket where I keep my wallet, when I heard the reassuring voice of Mr. Roberson. With a laugh he explained to me that his son was asking for a token for the vending machine. Arnold, was just exercising his rights as a patient of the office.

WHAT'S YOUR NAME?

THOUGH LOTHA WALLACE was less than three years old, she impressed people with her intelligence. She could respond without hesitation to questions addressed to her and enjoyed meaningful conversation. Her grandmother, Tessye, gave Lotha well-deserved adoration and love, which she accepted as her due. Lotha produced a delightful impression on me as well, and at the end of her visit, I gave her a large number of stickers and a big piece of candy.

Tessye looked at little Lotha and told her to thank her doctor for the generous present. Lotha turned toward me and, with a challenging attitude, loudly posed the question, "What is your name?"

"My name is Doctor Tsesis," I replied with appropriate professional dignity.

"Thank you, Tsesis," said Lotha in acknowledgment of my good deed.

14

TESTIMONIES OF LOVE

If a being from another planet were to come to earth for a brief visit and wanted in the shortest possible amount of time to understand the meaning of the expressions "to love" and "to be a human," one of the best places for him to study would be a busy pediatric office. Nowhere else on earth is such priceless human love concentrated into such a small space.

The visitor would see newborn children and their mothers and fathers treating these babies as if they were the most precious objects in the world; he would see healthy and sick children whose parents are caring for them, protecting them, forgiving them, comforting them, and cleaning them, totally oblivious to the unpleasant physiological functions of human beings. He would see tears and joy, anger and smiles, anxiety and bliss, and, most important, unconditional, dedicated, precious, all-absorbing, burning human love—a love in which a mother and father are not only ready, but happy to sacrifice their lives for the life and prosperity of their child.

LOVE WANTED

THE FAMOUS modern psychologist Erich Fromm stated in his still-popular book *The Art Of Loving* that love is a two-way street: for a true love relationship to exist between people, it is necessary that they have the capacity both to receive and to give love. One sign of a normal psyche is the desire to be loved by, and to give love to, other human beings.

I remember a story about the great French mathematician, astronomer, and physicist Pierre-Simon Laplace. On his deathbed, Laplace was attended by one of his closest friends, who, observing Laplace's morose appearance, told him that he should be proud of all the great discoveries he had given to humanity during his lifetime. Laplace was silent.

"Sir," said the friend, "your name has already become immortal. What did you miss in your life?"

"Love," Laplace answered.

I can't remember a time during the last twelve years when Mrs. Mildred Sagan did not accompany her daughter Jennifer to an appointment. Mrs. Sagan was an intelligent and bright woman. Her husband was the owner of several auto body shops. I had never met him—he had never come into the office with Jennifer or with her younger brother and older sister.

Jennifer was an exceptionally sensitive and charming sixteen-year-old young lady who had, as of late, become stupendously beautiful. She could easily have been chosen as a model of teenage beauty. Her face had classical features, and her skin was smooth and lustrous. She was tall, with a well-developed figure.

At first glance, Jennifer presented many of the signs of chronic fatigue syndrome: of late she had been depressed, lacked her usual energy, and was sleepy. Also, her academic performance had been poor.

A detailed history of the condition did not offer any clues to the cause of Jennifer's complaint, and the results of her physical examination were completely negative. The simple laboratory tests that I performed in the office were negative as well, and I told Mrs. Sagan that I did not think that the further laboratory workup she had requested at the beginning of the visit was going to add anything to help me in my diagnosis.

"In that case," she said, "I think I know why she is in such a melancholy mood. I am glad that she does not have any physical cause for her problem. We came to you to rule that out."

"Why didn't you tell me from the beginning that you knew the reason?" I asked.

I received no answer to this question, so I asked Mrs. Sagan to tell me what was behind Jennifer's lack of energy.

"I am in the process of getting a divorce from my husband," she answered. "He lives like a playboy. For the last several years he has come home at late hours, or sometimes not at all. I'm happy I've finally made the decision to divorce him; my other children feel the same way. Only Jennifer has taken it very hard. She was always her father's favorite: he always spent a lot of time with her when she was younger. Now he hardly speaks with her. I guess she misses him."

Further conversation with Jennifer confirmed her mother's concerns. Jennifer's feelings could be read on her open face. Unfortunately, she could not express herself in words; I tried to help her by asking some leading questions, which she was glad to answer.

I did not suggest anything extraordinary. I just recommended that Jennifer have a talk with her father, during which she should tell him not to forget about her, that he should spend at least a little time with her because she needed to see that he still loved her. For another ten minutes or so we discussed Jennifer's concerns and then parted.

I left the office with a heavy heart. I hoped that my patient would successfully resolve her problem, but at the same time I knew how unlikely it was that Mr. Sagan would be understanding and sensitive to his daughter's pain.

A week passed very quickly, and Jennifer returned for a follow-up visit. As soon as I entered the exam room, I saw that she had regained her usual appearance—she was contented and relaxed. A small miracle had happened after Jennifer spoke with her father. He did understand her emotional needs and promised to spend some special time with her. He was not too magnanimous—he promised only an hour or two a week—but Jennifer did not need more. Like a fish that cannot live when it is taken out of water, Jennifer could not live without the love that she had become used to since her infancy. All she needed was some reassurance from her father that he still loved her as much as he had in the good old times.

UNDER HER HEART

BOTH JANE O'CONNOR and her husband, Melvin, were serving in the U.S. Navy. At twenty-five Jane looked as if she had only just reached adulthood. Though she was attractive, she was not beautiful. Her appearance presented no example of classical beauty, and the skin of her face, which had probably never been touched by makeup, was not well cared for. She usually wore a pair of jeans and a baggy cotton shirt. To me, with whom she had a really friendly relationship, this apparent lack of femininity was more than compensated for by the remarkable warm glow that emanated from her kind hazel eyes.

Jane had grown up in a nearby suburb. After graduating from high school, she worked first as a clerk, then a secretary, and then a saleswoman, until one day she decided that her life needed a drastic change.

This happened about three years before I met her. She went to a local recruiting office and signed up with the navy. About a year and a half later she was serving as a petty officer in Naples, Italy, where she met Melvin. A year later they were married, and in due time their first child, Andrew, was born. Now Andrew, a patient of mine, was three months old.

Jane had taken a long leave from the service and had come home with her son for a two month visit. She was staying at the house in which she had grown up. Her family consisted of her parents and three siblings, but only her younger sister still lived at home. Her parents had been separated for a while and were residing in different states, while her older sister and brother were married and lived in their own apartments.

She had found out about my office from an old friend, and about a week after her arrival from Italy she had brought Andrew in for a visit. Since that visit Jane had brought her handsome and well cared for son in for several different minor health problems almost every other week. First, it was because Andrew was not gaining weight well, then it was for a mild respiratory infection, and then for a skin rash. Though it might appear to an outsider that Jane was being an overly cautious and protective mother, I knew that she really needed not just my professional support but my moral support as well—she could not expect it from her sister, who was six years younger than she, or from her husband and parents, with whom she communicated only by phone calls and letters. She needed some encouraging reassurance that her son was doing well.

Military life had evidently had a favorable influence on Jane— she brought to each visit good questions that had been carefully written out. She listened with real interest to my answers, writing notes in a small memo pad that she never forgot to bring with her.

Though Jane was a quiet person with a good self-image, at the end of her fourth visit something happened that was difficult for me to understand. Andrew had been brought in for a slight diaper rash. The rash was so minor that I thought it would be beneficial for Jane if I told her that she should not worry too much about trivial problems. To give more weight to my words, I concluded by telling her that most young mothers would not even pay attention to such a mild rash.

At this, unexpectedly, Jane became visibly upset, though I had provided my reassurance with the best intentions. I noticed a subtle, guilty smile on her face, and she was unable to look me in the eye.

While perplexed by the change in her behavior, I, nevertheless, continued to tell her how to take care of Andrew's sensitive skin. I handed her a prescription and a list of instructions and then asked her if she had any other questions. Jane took the hint and understood what was behind the emphatic and meaningful tone I had used with this last question. "I feel so awkward," she said in a low, but firm voice. "I'm afraid that in your eyes I must look stupid and inexperienced after coming into your office with my son so often."

As convincingly as I could, I told her that she was an excellent mother and that I could testify to that anytime. I added that if I was somewhat awkward during our conversation, she should forgive me, because I had never meant to imply that she was not a good caregiver. As she packed up her precious son, I proved to her, point by point, that she was a very loving and caring mother.

Finally she was done with her packing job. Holding Andrew against her chest with both arms, she gave him a look full of love and boundless admiration and then suddenly smiled generously at me. Her sincere voice then followed, which could have come from heaven rather than from her.

"Dr. Tsesis," this petty officer of the U.S. Navy and young parent Jane O'Connor said to me as she continued to press her precious baby to her chest, "how could I not be a good mother? I carried Andrew under my heart for nine long months!"

THE ABANDONED ANGEL

ANGEL TUTTON, an infant who had been under my care since she was born, was now four months old. Her appearance radiated health, and her skin shone with virtuous cleanliness. Her grandmother, Betsy Albright, was bustling around her on this day, trying, like any good artist, to put the finishing touches on her masterpiece, little Angel. Despite the reassuring manifestations of love and care that the child had been receiving, I was concerned because Angel had been accompanied to my office by her mother for only the first two visits; thereafter, she had always been brought in by her grandmother.

While looking at Angel's chart, I also discovered that Angel was now covered by public aid insurance, although for her first two months of life she had been covered by an HMO. Moreover, the public aid card was not issued in her mother's name but was under the name of Betsy Albright.

While Betsy was attending to Angel—not stopping for a moment in her whir of wiping this and changing that—I asked her why Angel's mother had not shown up for so long.

Betsy was silent, and I was forced to repeat my question. This time she responded. Interrupting her bustle around Angel, she, first hesitantly, then more willingly, told me that her daughter Hope did not live with her and Angel any longer.

She continued with a slight reproach in her voice. "She is twenty years old. You kept telling me during each visit that she, not I, should be actively involved in any discussion of her child's care. But, it was happening not because I am a chatterbox or a domineering mother but because I was the only one who was taking care of Angel—Hope was doing almost nothing and made no secret of it."

Naturally and without dramatization, Betsy told me the heart-breaking story of Angel's abandonment by her mother.

"Doctor, Hope was a very good girl; she graduated from high school with good grades and then began taking a couple courses at a local college. I was very proud of her."

Betsy paused, as if the pain of these recollections had struck her heart.

"Then she got involved with a local gang, and one of the gang members, Umberto, the one I hated most of all, became Angel's father. He introduced Hope to drugs and alcohol.

"Umberto, who was twelve years older than my daughter, had three children by another woman. When Angel was born, he said that he had a commitment to his previous children and that he could not take care of Angel as well because 'it was just too much for him.' Since Angel's birth he has not given a penny for the baby.

"Yes, Hope was a wonderful kid, but once she started with Umberto, I could hardly recognize her. Drugs made her absolutely different from the way she was before. She couldn't cope with the reality of life anymore. Rather than becoming more mature, she decided that she was going to enjoy her life no matter what it took or who suffered.

"To get the state to help, I was forced to apply to the public aid agency. They provided me with assistance, but they also initiated a lawsuit against my daughter for child abandonment. Hope shouldn't have done that."

After a short pause, Betsy, now sounding more like Hope's mother, added, "But if she was on drugs and alcohol, they should help her, right? I'm sure she would never have left her daughter if it wasn't for the cocaine.

"The last time she saw Angel was two months and two days ago when she visited our apartment. She didn't even kiss Angel. She lives somewhere with Umberto. She's never called me since."

To soften Betsy's unhappiness, I told her that something might have happened to Hope that had prevented her from coming back, but Betsy answered that different people who knew her daughter had seen Hope in the neighborhood since that time.

"Who helps you to take care of this little angel?" I asked Betsy, as she kissed Angel's fat and blooming cheeks.

"Oh, thank God, my sister helps me when I really need it. A month ago I had severe bronchitis, and without her help I don't know what would have happened to Angel. I couldn't even take care of myself at that time."

Trying to give Betsy some much needed encouragement, I praised her as an excellent grandmother and finished my consolation with a suggestion. "For practical reasons, you should try to obtain full guardianship over Angel."

"I am in the process of obtaining it," she answered, "In the meantime the court granted Hope the right to see Angel once a week for an hour, but she doesn't even want to do that."

Looking attentively at Betsy's face, I saw that she did not look well. She was short, and rather plump, her face was pockmarked, and her cheeks were starting to sag. The color of her face was yellowish, which was, without a doubt, due to her infrequent exposure to fresh air and sunshine.

Betsy, however, was far from being conquered. She considered herself to be a lucky grandmother who was privileged to be able to take care of her precious grandchild. Though her life was busy and tiring, she found deep meaning in taking care of her beloved Angel—meaning that her daughter was not looking for and, perhaps, would be unable to recognize.

For the future? In Betsy's situation it was too dangerous to think about the future. The present condition was enough for her to worry about, let alone worrying that something worse might happen at a future time. Didn't she already have more problems than one human being could carry? Had she not redeemed herself by becoming a mother to her granddaughter? The blissful expression on Angel's face, who was sucking on a pacifier with dedication, was enough to dispel grandma's worries.

I asked Betsy how old she was and could not believe what I heard: she was only fifty years old.

Trying to compliment her and lift her spirits, I told her that she looked much younger than her age. "Betsy, you look good. I am two years older than you, but you look ten years younger than I."

I did not think that my words would produce such an excited effect on Betsy. Addressing her grandchild in a lively and delighted voice, she exclaimed, "Did you hear that, Angel? I am younger than the doctor! Did you hear that!"

My assistant reminded me that there were other patients waiting for me. I had to go.

"Betsy, I'm very sorry that you should have to go through this misfortune when you are having problems with your own health."

Betsy looked at me with her amiable smile. I saw an expression of dedication on her face.

"Somebody has to do it, Doctor! Right?" she responded.

I agreed with her as I left the exam room. Meanwhile grandma Betsy began to dress Angel in her colorful clothes.

"You are such a good baby!" she said to her and then realized that her granddaughter was fast asleep.

"Oh, Angel, you don't even hear," she said, looking at her granddaughter's serene face.

"God bless Grandma's baby!" she exclaimed while picking up Angel, whose nose was sticking out from the pink package in which she was wrapped.

She repeated the last sentence several times and I joined her in her testimony of love.

MR. MOM

FEW PEOPLE can explain the reason they fall in love; even fewer can explain how they love. This was well expressed in the words of the French philosopher Blaise Pascal: "The heart has its reasons of which reason knows nothing."

This quotation came to mind when I met air-traffic controller Eric Smith, who came into my office for the first time with his sixteen-month-old son, Norman.

Before I had even spoken to Mr. Smith, I learned from the entries on Norman's chart that his parents were not married. Nothing unusual in that.

Bearing in mind the loss of many of the traditions that surround the family, it was still unusual that Norman's mother was not around. Usually the mother is present during a child's first visit to a new pediatrician.

Mr. Smith, a short but athletically built man, wore two-piece suit with a necktie. His confident movements as he prepared his son for his exam demonstrated that he was a person who knew the ropes of parenting.

I introduced myself and began to gather a comprehensive health history of the baby. At the end of the interview I asked Mr. Smith why Norman's mother had not come for this visit.

"Your girlfriend was busy today?" I asked.

Still busy bustling around his son, the father answered abruptly and without looking at me, "She is not my girlfriend."

"The mother of your son could not come because she is at work. Is my guess right?" I insisted.

"No, Doctor, you are wrong."

Two other guesses were wrong as well. Finally, Mr. Smith, seeing my unabated interest, lifted his eyes in my direction.

"If you really want to know, I'll tell you," he said, not displaying any enthusiasm.

I assured him that as a pediatrician, I needed to know the family relationships.

"She did not come because it was my turn to be with Norman. I alternate watching Norman with his mother. I work the night shift, so during the daytime every working day Norman is with me; the rest of the time he is with his mother, who is not working. I really don't know what she is doing with herself during the day; I am not interested."

I told Mr. Smith that though I deal daily with many families, such an arrangement was new to me; I asked him to give me more details about the relations between himself and his son's mother.

"I was dating his mother some two and a half years ago," Mr. Smith said, pointing his finger in his son's direction.

"For a while we were on good terms. Then about two years ago things started to fall apart between us. She became antagonistic and sarcastic toward me. We broke it off, forever, as I thought at the time.

"Early one morning around two-and-a-half months ago, I was leaving my work after my shift when I noticed a woman at the door calling me by my first name.

"Familiar voice, I thought to myself, and looked in her direction. Before me was Margaret, my former girlfriend. After the insults and humiliations I had taken from her, I didn't want to speak to her. Who wants to open a closed wound?

"I continued to walk as if she were not there, but she was following me.

"'What do you want from me?'" I turned and said, 'Just leave me alone!'"

"'I don't need anything from you,' she answered, 'but you might want to know that you have a son!'

"You see," Norman's father continued, "she knew my weak point. When we were on better terms, I had told her more than once that I wanted, someday, to have a child, a son. As she expected, that pushed my button."

"She asked me to come to her car, and there was Norman sitting in his car seat. Something inside me told me that he was my son, but my feelings toward Margaret were so suspicious that I was afraid she was trying to deceive me. In the end, we went for a very accurate genetic paternity test—it proved beyond a doubt that Norman was my child.

"Two weeks later, I began the process of officially becoming Norman's father under the law. And here he is!" he said, as he lifted up his happy child in his arms and carefully placed him back on the examining table.

"Why was it that you and Margaret were unable to reconcile and live together? You are a man with genuine human feelings. Does she not appreciate that?" I questioned.

"Forget it. She is much too childish for that. Norman could have had a father since the day he was born, but his mother's immaturity prevented her from letting me know that I had a child. Eventually, when Norman became thirteen months old, Margaret decided that it would be better for the child to have a father. Thank God for that! The minute I saw Norman, I fell in love with him. Don't ask me why. I don't know."

His son started to cry. Eric picked Norman up, fixed something about his shirt, offered him a drink from his bottle, and kissed his fat cheek.

"You are a regular Mr. Mom," I remarked, observing his dedication to taking care of his little Norman and the pleasure he got from it.

"People say that," Eric admitted.

MODESTY

MRS. BETTY YATES worked as a teller for the local bank. Her husband worked as a chef for a small catering company that he owned with his cousin. They were happily married and had three nice children, all of whom had been born during my tenure at my current office.

Betty, together with her own mother, brought a new patient in for a visit—two-week-old Aaron—a child that Betty and her husband had begun adoption proceedings on three days before.

To the novice, all newborn babies look alike. With experience it becomes possible to see the individuality of each separate child. Baby Aaron's face at his young age had an unforgettable appearance. He was a wonderfully cute baby with huge, alert eyes and a mass of tiny black ringlets above a wellshaped forehead.

Mrs. Yates, usually a cheerful, although a demure and quiet, person, was initially reluctant to tell me the details of this pending adoption. Gradually, over the course of the baby exam, I found out that Aaron had been born to Betty's sister, who was thirty years old, and who would never have given Aaron up for adoption if she had not been incarcerated for selling drugs. She had served five months of her sentence and had four years to go.

Little Aaron could be considered quite a lucky baby. In this time of the decline of the family, if his aunt or some other immediate family member had not been willing to take Aaron in, he would have become a part of the huge and ever-increasing state foster child care system.

When a mother is imprisoned, her child or children are punished as well—for the crime of their parent, not their own. Children, even very small children who really need to be with their mothers, are not a part of the penitentiary system, and this is just the reality of life.

Aaron, however, had the good luck to have a loving aunt and a family who were happy to share their food, shelter, and hearts with him.

The well-baby visit of a young child is one of the most pleasant parts of pediatric practice; at two weeks of age Aaron was healthy and very delightful—truly a cuddly gift from heaven. After giving some medical advice to the "new mother" and answering her questions, I told her that I thought it was wonderful that she and her husband had come to the rescue of this tender and helpless creature. Mrs. Yates only smiled bashfully in response. Mrs. Yates's mother, who was present in the exam room during the entire visit, was even less talkative than her daughter. Nevertheless, they both were friendly and appreciative.

I excused myself for a moment, went through my files, and brought back a poem by the American writer John Nay that had been given to me by one of my friends some time ago. I wanted Mrs. Yates to hear this verse.

"This is about you," I said to Betty:

How did he git thar? Angels.
  He could never have walked in that storm.
They jest scooped down and toted him
  To whar it was safe and warm.
And I think that saving a little child,
  And fotching him to his own,
Is a derned sight better business
  Than loafing around the Throne.

The visit was over, and we parted with a warm handshake. I left the room, while Betty and her mother, with a businesslike appearance, put their precious Aaron into his many layers of clothing.

The Yates were my last patients of the morning. As I took my new patient's chart to the reception desk, I noticed that the usually noisy waiting room was empty except for a dimly lighted corner where two toddlers—a boy and a girl—played happily with some toys as they spoke in soft voices. I looked around but was unable to see their parents. One of my receptionists was carefully watching them as if she were baby-sitting.

"Who are these kids?" I asked her in a perplexed tone.

"Oh, those are the children the Yates recently adopted," my receptionist answered, surprised that I had not learned this after spending more than half an hour with their new mother.

No, I knew nothing about these children. Betty had not mentioned anything about them. She had been too modest to tell me about the other two children, whose lives she was also trying to save for something meaningful and constructive.

If, as the poem said, to save one little child was such an exalted deed, how much greater was it to save three.

A MOTHER'S TEARS

THE FARNON family began coming to my office two years ago, when their first child was born. They were both in their early forties, mature and solid people. They had wanted to have a baby for many years and, having finally become parents, gave their daughter, Alison, all of the parental passion that they had accumulated during their long wait. Alison's mother, Laurie, was not beautiful; she was moderately overweight and had lost the grace of her past youth. Nevertheless, this impression was immediately dispelled after just a few minutes of conversation with her, especially when that conversation was about her firstborn—an internal light would then shine from her earnest, wide face, making her look attractive and young once again.

Laurie's husband, Steve, who was at least five years older than she, worked as a manager in a large department store. Like his wife, he was a decent and reliable person.

Given the conditions in which Alison was growing up, surrounded by constant, maybe even exaggerated parental love and attention, there could have been a great chance that Alison would come out spoiled and selfish, but, fortunately, such was not the case. She was born with a sense of humor and respect for others, which prevented her from becoming spoiled and made each encounter with her a real delight.

One day in November, Alison was brought to my office for a follow-up exam, and, as always, she was escorted by both her parents. Alison at two years of age weighed as much as a normal four-year-old. She was a tall, proportionately built, energetic girl. With a constant expression of mischief on her face, she was an embodiment of joie de vivre, or, as had been said of her by her father—she was a compact bundle of power.

Alison was a bundle of power of a pleasant kind—she would run swiftly back and forth in my office, but she would obediently follow her parents' request to stop. She never became wild during her activities; moreover, in the middle of a new prank, she would look at the people around her and smile charmingly at them, as if inviting them to join in her enthusiastic celebration of life.

During an exam, procedures that were unpleasant for Alison would make her cry and cause her to make all sorts of ugly facial expressions, but as soon as they were over, she would be back to her usual, joyful self.

Alison had been brought one day for conjunctivitis that she had developed two weeks earlier. I examined her the week before and gave the Farnons some eye drops for Alison, with the expectation that the condition would quickly improve. Unfortunately this had not happened, and the conjunctivitis persisted. My schedule for this day, which was light, gave me the time to carefully perform an eye examination. While I performed this exam, Mrs. Farnon observed me carefully and sometimes gave me an enigmatic smile.

Some parents tend to blame the doctor for the lack of improvement in their child's condition. When Laurie asked me something in a manner that I misunderstood as a polite reproach for the poor results of the previously prescribed treatment, I patiently and in minute detail explained my thoughts on the diagnosis and my plan for the treatment of what I now considered to be an allergic reaction to something, as yet unknown to me.

In order to determine the cause of this allergy, I asked the Farnons about Alison's environment.

Laurie's face brightened at this, and she turned to her husband and said, "I bet it's that rug, the one Alison plays on. I've wanted to throw it away many times because our cat used to sleep on it. The cat, which we don't have anymore, used to shed on this rug a lot."

I agreed with Laurie that the rug could be responsible for Alison's condition but then remarked that there might be other possible sources of allergy that she might not even suspect. With this, I handed the Farnons the medicine for allergic conjunctivitis, and they left the exam room. Their daughter, who was producing all kinds of funny sounds as she continuously flashed her beautiful smile, led the way.

Alison's appointment was my last of the morning. After quickly finishing with my paperwork, I left the office and got in my car to go to lunch. It was unusually warm for this time of year, so I opened the windows. I backed up and was ready to leave when I noticed a solitary couple across the street, who were embracing one another. This was an unusual sight and I looked at them closely until, to my surprise, I realized that this couple was Mr. and Mrs. Farnon.

I drove toward them, and as the car approached, I realized that it was, indeed, Laurie embracing her husband as they stood next to their car. She was sobbing on Steve's shoulder while, packed inside the car, their "bundle of power" was entertaining herself.

Alarming thoughts immediately filled my mind. Had I inadvertently said something offensive to Laurie, Steve, or their daughter? Had someone on my staff insulted the family?

Mr. Farnon then noticed me, gently moved Laurie aside, and walked toward me as I remained seated in my car. I waited with some degree of nervousness for what he was going to say.

Laurie's red cheeks were wet with the tears that still ran from her eyes, but I noticed an apologetic smile on Steve Farnon's face that signaled to me that I was not the cause of Laurie's distress.

"My wife just does not take things well," Steve said to me as he got closer to my car, "so I'm trying to comfort her."

Although he did not actually invite me to help him out with his wife, I understood that he would not mind if I tried. If I was not the reason for Laurie's distress, then what was? I gave Laurie a questioning look as she walked toward me, wiping her eyes in a childlike manner with her right fist. I wanted to get out of the car but was prevented both by Steve, who was standing in front of the door, and by the tension of the moment.

Steve and I waited for Laurie to speak, but she remained silent. "It's Alison's eyes, Doctor," she finally said. "I feel so bad about it. I should have thought of that rug before all this happened. I did wonder if it might be the reason for Alison's problems and wanted to throw it away, but I just put it off."

Then, as if continuing the conversation with her husband that had caused her to cry, she said, "Do you think this might have happened because we had Alison so late?"

She stopped for a second and then resumed. "Do we give Alison all she needs? Maybe we should have more children? But we are old." She answered her own question, and her tears again began to run.

I understood that Laurie was trying to resolve issues that had concerned her for a long time. She was a typical mother, who would always feel an infinite responsibility toward her child, a mother for whom loving her child came as naturally as breathing. Any amount of love that she could provide to Alison did not seem like enough to her. The guilt that she could not provide endless love tormented her heart. Looking at her, I could see the devotion and kindness in her eyes, a love that cannot be obtained by all the gold in the world.

What could I tell her? How could I put her mind at ease without running the risk of appearing false and artificial? How could I put some thousands of words into only a few?

Without realizing what I was doing, I jumped out of my car and took her right hand, still wet with tears, into mine.

I brought her hand to my face and tightly pressed it to my lips. As I looked at her face, I understood that there was no need for words. Our hearts had spoken for us.

Two weeks later, Alison was brought in again by her devoted chaperons. As usual, Alison was happy as a lark, creating minor storms and whirlwinds around her. Her parents were happy as well: Alison's allergic conjunctivitis had completely gone.

Laurie's guess was correct. Probably her maternal intuition had helped her to figure out what had caused her daughter's allergy.

WITH CHILDREN IN MIND

EVEN IN this time of equality between the sexes, mothers continue to be the central figure in the physical, mental, and emotional nurturing of children. As during the prior years of humanity's history, the overwhelming majority of mothers are unconditionally devoted to their offspring. Over the years I have observed a common phenomenon: the mind of a mother, especially the mother of a younger child, perceives the world through her prism of concerns, worries, and apprehensions about her children.

Lucy Serritella had brought her children to my office for at least seven years before I joined the practice. Since my arrival at this practice, in addition to the growth and blossoming of her three children, I had been an eyewitness to the many changes in her life as well. She had divorced her husband; I had mistakenly thought that they got on well together before this divorce. After the divorce she had lost weight—at least 100 pounds—transforming herself from a tall, stout woman to a slim beauty. She also changed from being a well-to-do housewife to being a very successful business administrator.

In the twelve years I had known Lucy, however, two things had not changed—her forthright character and the unique beauty of her refined, aristocratic, delicate face.

As I examined her twelve-year-old daughter, she unexpectedly asked me what country I had come from.

"Will you go back to see your home and your old friends?" she asked me, after I told her that I was from Russia.

"No," I replied. "I do not want to go back to the country where I was not respected as a human being."

"I can understand this," Lucy remarked. "With three children, I sometimes feel the same way."

Bernice Morgan, an energetic, friendly, and young-looking woman who was an experienced saleswoman, was also the mother of two sons and two daughter. Ever since I met her, I have enjoyed her sense of humor.

While examining her one-year-old son, I noticed that he had an unusually large forehead. I looked at Bernice and realized that her forehead was large as well—only in her case it had not been as noticeable because she wore her hair in bangs, which hid her generous forehead.

"Bernice, I never realized before that your forehead is so large. I bet you are very talented at your work. They say that geniuses frequently have large foreheads because they need them to hold all those brains."

Bernice chuckled and corrected me. "I don't know about my work, but, of course, I am a genius. That's why I have four children."

ENJOYING LOVE

FIFTEEN-MONTH-OLD Marcos Weber had taken his vaccinations like a man.

Ten minutes later when, with his short memory, all recollection of the unpleasantness had gone, he once again resumed his main activity—the enjoyment of life. His mother, who was all dressed up, as she had just come from work, had been softly comforting him and was ready to begin dressing him.

Marcos was standing on the edge of the examining table, opposite his mother, chirping something in his own language and bouncing up and down like a spring. To the outside observer it would have appeared that the son and the mother were involved in a lively conversation.

Mrs. Weber pulled out a fresh diaper from the diaper bag and was ready to put it on Marcos. At that moment her son, who was still cheerfully explaining something of great importance to his mother, produced a graceful, strong arc of urine from his little spigot straight onto his mother's lovely blouse.

Mrs. Weber, who evidently enjoyed motherhood and all that comes with it, patiently stood in front of her energetically peeing boy—she did not dare to interrupt her son's bodily function.

As her blouse quickly became soaked with her son's natural juice, she looked at her beloved son with eyes full of love and adoration and, smiling broadly, said again and again in a pseudosarcastic tone, each time adding more maternal tenderness to it, "Thanks a lot, son! Thanks a lot."

SHAWN PARKER HAS INFECTIOUS MONO

PARENTS ARE their children's keepers. The mind of every devoted parent is focused on the protection and well-being of their offsprings.

Shawn, a ten-year-old, presented complaints typical of infectious mononucleosis, or mono in laypersons' terms: he was tired, and feverish, and had a sore throat, and the glands in his neck were enlarged.

From previous experience I knew that Shawn's mother, Mrs. Parker, was probably afraid that her son had a malignant disease such as leukemia, which could be associated with symptoms similar to those that her son now showed. To prove my clinical diagnosis of mono, I ordered two tests to be performed in the office: a complete blood count and another test that was more specific for mono, a monospot test.

The results of the complete blood count came first and confirmed, though not directly, my clinical diagnosis; the number of white blood cells, especially of the lymphocytic variety, were increased. I tried to explain to Shawn's mother why this result pointed to mono. Mrs. Parker, however, a quiet, stable, and intelligent woman whom I had known for a long time, had obviously read some medical literature and had heard the "enlightened" opinions of her relatives before she had brought her son in. Thus, all of this intimidating information had so badly frightened her that she was unable to accept my reassurances.

I decided to wait for the second study, the monospot test; if positive, it would firmly establish the diagnosis. I thought that with a precise and unambiguous result it would be much easier to persuade

Mrs. Parker that her son was not in any danger.

The result of the monospot test came in about ten minutes; as I had expected, it was positive. A big, clear-cut "plus" sign on the white background of the slide left no uncertainty as to Shawn's diagnosis.

It is pleasant to have an exact diagnosis of an illness. It allows the physician to provide appropriate treatment and helps in determining the prognosis for the condition as well. For Shawn, who had a mild to moderate form of "mono," no treatment was necessary. The tincture of time was the best healer for him. His prognosis was excellent.

Thinking that I could now easily reassure Mrs. Parker, I could not resist the temptation of producing the external evidence—I brought the slide with the positive result with me so that Shawn's mother could see it with her own eyes.

Mrs. Parker, who was still under the stress of expecting bad news, first looked at the offered slide and then at me. Her eyes were open wide, but she said nothing.

"What do you see there?" I asked her with an encouraging smile. Her response was minimal.

She looked fixedly at the slide, visibly becoming more nervous and anxious. Suddenly a sharp pain distorted her usually serene face, and with horror in her voice she loudly exclaimed, "Oh, my God! A cross! I see a cross!"

The rest of the visit was spent in reassuring Mrs. Parker that her son's condition was benign. Eventually, she began to hear what I was telling her and understood that her son did not suffer from any serious condition.

Three days later, when Shawn came in with his mother for a follow-up visit, the child was in much better shape than he had been previously. By now his fatigue, fever, sore throat, and enlarged glands were all in the past. His mother was also much improved; she had forgotten her dark premonitions and terrible expectations and was in her usual optimistic mood.

PARENTAL GENEROSITY

GREGORY RANDOLF was a sixteen-year-old with a common problem for his age—acne. Acne, or "zits," of different colors and shapes covered his forehead, cheeks, and chin in abundance. Gregory was a friendly and cooperative teenager.

His mother, Mona Randolf, was present with him in the exam room. It was Gregory's third visit for his skin condition, and Mona had brought along all of his medications, contained in several vials and tubes, which she neatly placed on my desk.

Beyond a doubt, Gregory had been very compliant with the medical regimen that had been prescribed for him by me, but, unfortunately, his numerous, deep-seated cysts were not responding to the treatment, which consisted of an oral antibiotic and topical creams and wipes.

On this visit it became clear to me that he was a candidate for treatment with a relatively new medication—Accutane®. Accutane® is a derivative of vitamin A. This medication produces a miraculous, long-lasting effect in a significant number of acne patients. Alas, there is no such thing as a free lunch—this medication has several serious drawbacks: it is tremendously teratogenic for pregnant women, and it may produce changes, sometimes even, though rarely, irreversible changes, in numerous bodily organs and systems. Therefore, it is prescribed to patients, especially to young women, only with extreme caution. Patients who are taking Accutane® should be carefully monitored by clinical observation and laboratory tests.

This, together with the prohibitively high cost of the medicine, brings the total expense for the full course of treatment to an amount that is around $1,000.

Both Mrs. Randolf and her son were dressed in clean, but modest clothes; after the visit Mrs. Randolf usually paid immediately in cash, not waiting for the bill to come by mail—she did not like to owe money to anybody. The Randolf family belonged to the lower middle class, lower to such a degree that they could not afford to buy health insurance. The expense of Gregory's treatment would, therefore, come out of their own pockets.

With enthusiasm I told the Randolfs about the possible positive effect of Accutane treatment for Gregory, who was being affected emotionally by the ugly pimples on his face. The enthusiasm was gone from my voice when I enumerated the drawbacks associated with the treatment with Accutane®. When I concluded with the $1,000 price tag associated with the treatment, my voice fell to a whisper.

But Mrs. Randolf was dedicated to provide complete protection for her son's health and physical appearance, even if this health condition was not life-threatening.

This simple, unsophisticated woman gave a brief look at her son. At this instant, I could see in her eyes infinite love and devotion for Gregory. Without a trace of hesitation and with a tender smile on her face she said, "It's Ok. He well deserves it."